1998

OXFORD MEDICAL PU

D0383397

TOURETTE SYNDROME

the**facts**

the**facts**

ALSO AVAILABLE IN THE SERIES

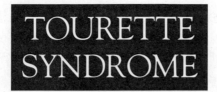

TOURETTE SYNDROME

the**facts**

Second Edition

Mary M Robertson
Department of Psychiatry,
and Behavioural Sciences
University College London Medical School

and

Simon Baron-Cohen
Departments of Experimental Psychology
and Psychiatry
University of Cambridge

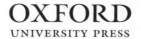

OXFORD
UNIVERSITY PRESS

OXFORD

UNIVERSITY PRESS

Great Clarendon Street, Oxford OX2 6DP

Oxford University Press is a department of the University of Oxford.
It furthers the University's objective of excellence in research, scholarship,
and education by publishing worldwide in

Oxford New York

Auckland Bangkok Buenos Aires Cape Town Chennai
Dar es Salaam Delhi Hong Kong Istanbul Karachi Kolkata
Kuala Lumpur Madrid Melbourne Mexico City Mumbai Nairobi
São Paulo Shanghai Singapore Taipei Tokyo Toronto

and an associated company in Berlin

Oxford is a registered trade mark of Oxford University Press
in the UK and in certain other countries

Published in the United States
by Oxford University Press Inc., New York

Library of Congress Cataloging in Publication Data
Robertson, Mary M.
Tourette syndrome / Mary M. Robertson and Simon Baron-Cohen.
p. cm.—(Oxford medical publications) (The facts)
1. Tourette syndrome. I. Baron-Cohen, Simon. II. Title.
III. Series. IV. Series: The facts (Oxford, England)
[DNLM: 1. Tourette Syndrome. WM 197 R651t 1998]
RC375.R63   1998   616.8'3—dc21   97–18413

ISBN 0 19 852398 X

Printed in Great Britain
on acid-free paper by
Biddles Ltd., Guildford and King's Lynn

Preface

Over the years hundreds of children and adults with Tourette syndrome, and their families, have attended our clinic at the National Hospital, Queen Square, in London. They have repeatedly told us of their need for a readable, slim text on Tourette syndrome, summarizing what is known about the condition for a general reader; hence this book. We have not included references in the text, so as to keep this publication as user-friendly as possible. Jargon has been reduced to a minimum. Where terminology is needed, we have defined it. For those who wish to delve further into the large literature on this subject, a bibliography is provided at the end. We hope that patients and their families, many of whom have helped us considerably in our research, will find this book of value.

London   M.M.R.
September 1997   S.B-C.

Praise for **Tourette syndrome: the facts**

This excellent book manages to give a concise, balanced, practical and remarkably comprehensive discussion of almost all the questions and problems which children with Tourette's syndrome and their parents may face. In addition, there is a wide-ranging bibliography for those who wish to pursue the subject further, and a list of Tourette syndrome associations and interested physicians throughout the world. It is a most valuable resource.

Oliver Sacks

Tourette syndrome: the facts provides valuable up-to-date information not only for families who may be touched by this disorder, but also for both the general reader and medical professional. The authors use a unique approach in order to bridge the gap in interest between the lay and professional reader. By presenting typical and very human case histories the reader's interest is held as he moves along rapidly through well elucidated explanations of brain function and treatment complexities. We welcome this fine addition to the literature on this little known and poorly understood neurological condition.

Sue Levi-Pearl, Director
Medical & Scientific Programs
Tourette Syndrome Assoc., Inc. (US)

The Tourette Syndrome (UK) Association fully endorses the views expressed in the book . . . Indeed, a book such as this, which addresses all aspects of the disorder in a way that can easily be understood by the layperson, has been needed for some time. It will undoubtedly become the primary source of information, not just for those health and other professionals seeking a comprehensive introduction to the subject, but also a source of inspiration to many sufferers and their families.

Iain Steedman
General Secretary
Tourette Syndrome (UK) Association

Acknowledgements

We would like to thank the staff at Oxford University Press for their guidance in preparing this book. In addition, we are grateful to the Tourette Syndrome Associations in the UK and USA, and the NHS Anglia and Oxford Trust for supporting our research. Amber Carroll, Sue Levi-Pearl, Anne Mason, Paula Smith, and Drs Roger Freeman, Justin Livingston, and Kenneth Rickler read drafts of this book and gave us valuable suggestions for improving it, which we much appreciate. Shelagh Eggo skilfully revised the text and facilitated the whole process of writing the book. Trinity College Library kindly supplied Figure 5, and Peter Brooke generously sent us Figure 4. Finally, we are indebted to John Ludgate and Bridget Lindley for their support and encouragement at every level.

Illustrations

The figures in this book were reproduced by kind permission of the following sources:

Figure 1: Raven Press. *Advances in Neurology*, Volume 58.
Figures 2 and 3: Springer-Verlag, Heimer, L. *The Human Brain and Spinal Cord* (1983).
Figure 4: Maurice Benichou, L'homme Qui, Centre International de Creations Theatrales, Paris.
Figure 5: by Joshua Reynolds, reproduced from *Samuel Johnson* by John Wain (1974), MacMillan London, Ltd.

the**facts**

CONTENTS

1
Introducing three cases

Gilles de la Tourette syndrome (also known as Tourette's disorder, or Tourette syndrome for short) has been recognized as a medical condition for over 150 years. The main features include multiple *motor tics* (involuntary movements), and one or more *vocal or phonic tics* (noises) which occur in bouts many times a day. The number, frequency, and complexity of the tics often change over time. They can be quite mild in some cases (more like facial and vocal 'habits' or 'mannerisms' such as excessive blinking or squinting and repetitive sniffing) but these symptoms in others can be very distressing and disabling, interfering with one's actions and speech.

The first clear description of the syndrome was made in France in 1825, when Itard documented the case of a noblewoman, the Marquise de Dampierre. Subsequently, in 1885, the French neurologist and neuropsychiatrist Georges Gilles de la Tourette (Figure 1) working at the Salpetriere Hospital in Paris described nine cases of the syndrome, emphasizing the triad of multiple tics, coprolalia (inappropriate and involuntary swearing), and echolalia (involuntary echoing back of the speech of others).

Originally Tourette Syndrome was thought to be a rarity. For example, between 1825 and 1900 there were only 23 papers published on the topic in the medical literature, the majority of which were case reports. An international registry published in 1973 reported only 485 cases worldwide. Since then, however, the literature has expanded enormously, and substantial numbers of patients are now documented.

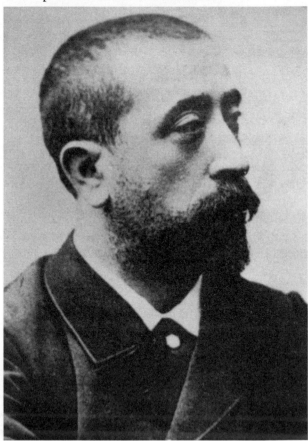

Figure 1 Gilles de la Tourette. Reprinted with permission from *Advances in Neurology*, 58. Raven Press, New York.

Tourette syndrome can take many forms. For some people it may involve mild facial tics and odd vocalizations. For others it involves more dramatic uncontrollable movements, and for a minority, involuntary swearing. In other cases, symptoms may be accompanied by additional problems such as overactivity, poor attention, and obsessions. Because of this broad range of expression, we begin by describing three cases of people with Tourette syndrome, each of whom is typical but in a different way. Naturally we have used fictitious names for them. In addition, these descriptions represent a combination of patients we have seen in our clinic, rather than specific people. Let us introduce you to them.

Johnny Thompson—a little volcano

Peggy and Peter Thompson were happily married. Peggy was an excellent, dedicated teacher who had a flair not only for imparting information to children, but also for bringing out the best in them. She loved her pupils and they, in turn, loved her. Peter was a successful lawyer and a partner in a large, prestigious practice specializing in patent law. Their only daughter, Laura, looked as though she was going to follow in her parents' footsteps. She was pretty, bright, popular at school, and succeeded not only in her studies, but also at her extra-curricular activities and hobbies. She was, in fact, almost the perfect child. Life in the Thompson household was idyllic. The atmosphere in the home was warm and happy.

Peggy and Peter had wanted another child for some time. They had tried and tried, but eventually after several doctor's consultations, Peggy was diagnosed as having 'secondary infertility'. Nevertheless, they were not put off, and kept on trying to have another child. After a couple of years they were delighted to discover that Peggy was pregnant. As Peggy was over 35 years old, an amniocentesis was recommended by the doctors, and, to everyone's relief the results were completely normal. Similarly, Peggy had a scan— and again it was, thankfully, normal. On the scan it was clear that the baby was a boy, and even during the pregnancy the parents called him Johnny.

Johnny made himself known early on. Even during pregnancy he was on the go all the time like a little volcano. He kicked, and kicked, and kicked. Peggy's initial dreams of Johnny representing England at rugby were soon replaced by her dreams for peace and quiet. At last the ninth month arrived, but after two weeks, Peggy went into premature labour. The delivery was assisted by forceps, apparently because Johnny was struggling despite his small size.

Peggy was sure Johnny was struggling because he was in too much of a rush: he just had to be born quickly! As soon as he arrived, Johnny began to cry— not gentle cries, but yells, as if to tell the world that he had arrived. Johnny continued to cry for what seemed like years. He cried during the day, but seemed to cry especially loudly at night, when others were trying to sleep. 'The crying drives me to hell and back', Peggy said to a close friend. Johnny didn't sleep at night or take afternoon naps, he screamed for hours on end, hated being held, and would struggle to be put down.

However, despite these initial problems, Johnny did seem to grow and mature at a normal rate. He ate well, but failed to put on much weight. The doctor suggested that there was really nothing wrong, and theorized that the lack of weight gain was probably because Johnny was never still, and was therefore using up too much energy. He moved constantly in his cot, in his pram, and even in his high-chair. At night he seemed to move all the time, leaving his cot in a mess in the morning, with the sheets all over the place. He also managed to bang his head in his sleep at night, which worried Peggy. Nevertheless, the family doctor continued to be reassuring; he said that many babies behaved like that, and that Peggy need not worry. She tried not to.

As a toddler Johnny had temper tantrums up to three or four times a day. He would throw things and break them and would try to hurt himself by banging his head on the floor or walls. The trigger for these rages was often something trivial, such as putting on the wrong shoe first.

By the time Johnny reached the age of the 'terrible twos', things were no better, but no worse. He made Peggy feel desperate. Peter was very supportive, but there was very little that he could do. Johnny was irritable, impatient, demanding, and couldn't take no for an answer. Life was exhausting. Laura, the older child, felt left out because so much attention was given to Johnny, but being such a placid and kind little girl, she accepted everything and seemed to continue to grow into a lovelier child.

The years went by. Johnny learned to talk: the only trouble was that he never seemed to stop talking, and he spoke in a very loud voice. He would butt into others' conversations, with no apparent regard for what they were saying.

When he started nursery school, it was also a disaster, unlike the peace of Laura's time there. Johnny drove the teachers to despair. Not only was he talkative, loud, intrusive, and even deafening at times, but he was also continually on the go. He had boundless energy. He had to hurry wherever he went.

He had never crawled and now he didn't walk—he seemed to run and dash everywhere. He climbed onto things, jumped into things, and, in his haste, seemed to act without thinking . At junior school things got even worse. He was unable to concentrate, he would sit gazing into space as if dreaming, not responding when spoken to. He would ask teachers to repeat what they had said. Johnny did not seem to understand instructions, and thus started falling behind at school.

Things got so bad that Peggy took Johnny back to the family doctor. The doctor knew the family well and he appreciated that both Peggy and Peter were sensible, good parents. He also knew that they had been a happy, uncomplicated family—until Johnny's arrival. The doctor found himself at a loss. Normally, when a child seemed so badly behaved, he would ask himself whether the problems might be the result of bad parenting or family troubles. In this family he knew that this was not the case. All he could do was reassure Peggy that it was part of 'growing up', and that, hopefully, Johnny would grow out of his awful behaviour.

But Johnny did not improve. Both at school and at home Johnny would make friends, but lose them as soon as they got to know him. He became isolated and lonely. Life was not a pleasure for anyone in the family any more. Johnny's behaviour began to get everyone down.

At about the age of eight, Johnny started to shake the hair out of his eyes excessively, and blow his fringe. These activities persisted and became labelled as 'habits'. His hair was rather long, so Peggy took him to the barber to have it cut. The haircut made no difference—he continued to flick his head and blow, even though his hair was now short. Then he began to screw up his eyes. The family doctor examined them and said that there were no problems with his sight.

Soon after, he began to stick out his tongue. Peggy and Peter reprimanded him, but that seemed to make matters worse. He not only stuck out his tongue, but also began to grimace. He also started both to smell and lick things, and occasionally he would spit—even in public. Life with Johnny was a continuous nightmare.

The family doctor was again consulted and this time he referred Johnny and the family to a child psychologist. The psychologist listened carefully, and, at the end of three assessment visits was only able to say that she had never come across a child like this. The psychologist raised the idea that there could be some family problems causing Johnny's behaviour. Peggy and Peter despaired. The next two years seemed to be full of constant noise and activity, with Johnny rushing about, apparently without thinking, not coping at school, having temper tantrums, and becoming lonelier.

Next Johnny began to repeat words and phrases he heard on TV, and would also repeat his own sentences or the last word of a sentence. He seemed distressed about his own behaviour, even though, to others, it seemed deliberate. Peggy couldn't win; disciplining him didn't seem to help, and ignoring the behaviour (in case it was just attention-seeking) didn't help either. She even thought it could be caused by a food allergy, so she didn't allow him to have sugar, dairy products, red food colouring or any food or drink with 'E' additives. Still his behaviour remained unchanged.

At the age of ten, Johnny started coughing and making strange noises in his throat, as if it needed clearing constantly. Peggy took him to the family doctor again. This time he referred Johnny to a paediatrician.

The paediatrician took one look at Johnny, took a brief history of the case, and pronounced that Johnny had Tourette syndrome with attention deficit hyper-activity disorder, also known as ADHD. Peggy and Peter had never heard of such a condition, but when the paediatrician explained it to them, things began to fall into place. Only when the paediatrician enquired carefully and specifically into the family history did Peter remember that his father used to clear his throat constantly, and that his brother used to twitch his nose. The family had affectionately called this his 'rabbit twitch'. Both men were happily married, successful in their careers and seemingly normal. Their noises and twitches were so much part of them, and they were such likeable people, that the 'symptoms' had never really been considered abnormal.

Tourette syndrome: at last Peggy and Peter had a name for Johnny's problems—and, with the diagno-sis, hopefully some help. The paediatrician had only seen a couple of cases of Tourette syndrome but had seen many more children with ADHD. He decided to try Johnny on some medication—methylphenidate (Ritalin). It seemed to be magic for the hyperactivity (which decreased) and the poor concentration (which improved). However, the tics and noises became much worse, and Johnny also began to lose weight. Nevertheless, because the ADHD and schoolwork improved, the paediatrician decided that this medication was better than nothing, and that Johnny should remain on it.

After another two years Johnny began to say 'fu, fu' and cough afterwards. Then, one day, he said the full, dreaded 'F word' in school assembly, and was clearly upset at having done so. The family made an immediate appointment to see the same paediatrician, who recognized that the Tourette syndrome was worsening, despite the methylphenidate. He made enquiries in the medical world, and decided to refer Johnny and the family to a specialist in Tourette syndrome. The specialist had seen hundreds of both children and adults with the syndrome, which reassured Peggy and Peter at once.

He took Johnny off methylphenidate as it may have increased the tics and noises, and prescribed clonidine instead. Johnny's tics and noises slowly improved, the swearing became less frequent and his concentration and hyperactivity remained under control. Life was never going to be easy with Johnny, but at least he was manageable. He began to catch up at school and even seemed to make some friends.

The specialist put the family in touch with the Tourette Syndrome Association (TSA), from which Peggy and Peter derived great comfort. They realized that their story was not so unusual, that Johnny was not a bad child; rather, he was a child in need of professional help, care, and understanding.

Now let's look at a different case of Tourette syndrome.

Tim–the teacher

Tim had had twitches and habits as long as he could remember. At five years old, when he had just started school, he began to blink a lot and roll his eyes. He soon began to have head nodding movements as well, which earned him the nickname of Noddy. At first his classmates teased him, and a few tried to bully him, but as he was temperamentally a fighter he never let this get him down.

Tim came from an ordinary and happy home. His grandfather ran a small family business selling kitchen hardware. His parents were healthy and rarely visited doctors. Both his father and grandfather had had facial twitches and made repetitive throat-clearing noises when under stress. His father also said that when he had been at school himself, he had had problems with concentration. However, his intelligence was above average and he was a hard worker which more than compensated for his occasional day dreaming. Tim had a brother and two sisters, all of whom had no serious problems in their lives.

Tim liked school. He enjoyed learning, acquiring knowledge, and his ambition was to become a teacher when he grew up. The nickname 'Noddy' stayed with him through junior school where, after some initial problems with teasing and bullying, the name became a term of endearment. He was a likeable child and got on with most of the other children. When he was 13 he developed a strange tickling feeling in his throat, and he felt compelled to clear his throat quite a lot. He remembered thinking that he did not have a sore throat and he did not have a temperature or feel ill, so it felt even stranger that he cleared his throat. Soon after that he began to cough for no good reason, and this became a habit. Occasionally when he coughed more than usual, people would ask him if he was coming down with a cold or flu, but he always replied that he was fine.

Tim's tics and noises became a part of him. He was certainly aware of them. Before a tic he would feel a tension, a tightness or a tickle in the area of the tic. He could stop the tics voluntarily, though this sometimes caused more inner tension. When this tension mounted up too much there seemed to be a rebound increase in tics after periods of controlling his symptoms. Tim's tics waxed and waned—sometimes they were more or less obvious—but this seemed to be for no apparent reason. If he developed flu or a fever his tics did seem to disappear temporarily. The tic pattern would also change at times, with old tics disappearing and new ones developing.

He also had an urge to imitate or copy what other people said or did, especially people on television programmes. He imitated people's accents, words, and mannerisms. Eventually, these copied behaviours became part of his own behaviour, so that he was like a tic-chameleon, absorbing and then reflecting the habits and noises of his surroundings. No one seemed to mind and it didn't bother Tim. In fact, mimicking became one of his party pieces, and a part of his developing character. At times he felt an urge to lick or smell things, but he realised the embarrassment this might create, so he was able to control the urge until he was alone. Then, he would smell or lick anything in sight.

Tim was above average academically, and did well at school. He was also good at sport, particularly soccer, and it was remarkable that his symptoms disappeared without any effort when he concentrated on sport. He went on to graduate from teacher training college, and began to teach at the age of 22.

Occasionally Tim liked to enjoy a pint of beer or glass of wine. He also had the odd puff of marijuana. Both the alcohol and the marijuana reduced the severity of his tics, but as his tics didn't really bother him, he was never tempted to use these substances to excess. Tim had always had friends and girlfriends. His first serious girlfriend, called Alison, was another junior teacher at the school. After dating seriously for nine months they decided to get married.

Tim was in his third year of teaching when Paul, a new nine year old pupil, arrived in his class. Paul was a bright child, but difficult to manage as he was constantly on the go, jumping up and down in class, interrupting, and talking excessively. At times Paul was very inattentive. Tim noticed that, like himself, Paul had some facial 'habits', and made little noises such as sniffing. He thought this was strange since apart from himself, his father and grandfather, Tim had never really noticed facial mannerisms in other people. Paul proved to be a real handful in class.

Shortly after this, Tim and the school headmaster received letters from a doctor who provided a medical description of Paul. Paul's facial twitches, habits, and sniffing noises were described as being part of Tourette syndrome, and his hyperactivity was part of an associated condition called attention deficit hyperactivity disorder (or ADHD). Paul had been put on medication and the school was given strategies on how to deal with him. Tim asked his family doctor if he could be referred to the hospital himself, not because he needed or wanted treatment, but because he was curious about the apparent similarities (tics and noises) and differences between himself and Paul. The specialist met, interviewed and examined Tim. He was indeed diagnosed as having Tourette syndrome, but it was so mild and Tim was so well-adjusted, that no medication was recommended.

Now let's look at our third and final case:

Jessie's story

Jessie Davis was a very special child. She was the only child born to parents in their forties. The pregnancy was normal apart from the fact that her mother, Kathy, was ill with excessive vomiting. The labour was normal in length, but Kathy was disappointed when forceps had to be used to assist in Jessie's birth. As a baby Jessie was very well-behaved. She smiled early, much to the delight of Kathy and her husband Frank. Her early development was normal; she seemed to sit, crawl, walk, and talk at the same time as other children of her age.

Jessie went to nursery school at three and managed the separation from her parents without fuss or distress. She was a naturally good mixer and particularly enjoyed playing with other children of her own age. She loved drawing, climbing on the jungle-gym, learning the alphabet, playing with plasticine, and doing sums. She laughed happily with her friends and when she went home in the afternoon she recounted her tales of fun to her mother.

Kathy was a part-time secretary. Her employer, a lawyer, valued her greatly as she was extremely well organized and a perfectionist. She was able to accomplish in one morning what a lot of people would have done in a day. Kathy ran her household with the same degree of precision. The home was decorated tastefully and well, all in pastel colours. Curtains and cushions were in the same fabric, ornaments were symmetrically organized and everything had its place. There were always fresh flowers in the dainty vase on the dining table, and the wooded floor shone so much that it seemed clean enough to eat off! Frank was an architect. Although he was not as neat and tidy as Kathy, he appreciated her liking things arranged neatly and symmetrically.

After a successful two years at nursery school, Jessie began primary school. A bright child and still a good mixer, she adapted well once again. She was well above her peers academically and proved to be a good all-rounder. When she was seven years old, Jessie's class teacher noticed that she would squint and blink her eyes excessively. The teacher told Kathy of Jessie's eye problem. Jessie's health had been good so far and Kathy was shocked to hear of a potential problem. Jessie seemed relatively unconcerned and reassured her mother that she felt no pain in her eyes. Nevertheless, Kathy was concerned, so the family doctor was consulted and he suggested that soothing eye drops should be put into Jessie's eyes three times a day. Kathy did as the doctor had said but it made no difference. Jessie did not seem particularly bothered, but her parents were worried.

Kathy made an appointment for Jessie to see an eye specialist. He put Jessie through all the usual tests, such as looking into her eye with an ophthalmoscope, examining her eyes through a slit lamp and getting her to read from a wall-chart. At the end of the examination, he said that Jessie's eyes and sight were normal and there was no need to worry.

The school holidays began and soon Kathy noticed that Jessie was blinking less often. When school started again it seemed as though the eye blinking had disappeared, but this behaviour was replaced by a stretching movement of Jessie's neck, as though her collar was too tight. Jessie said she felt a kind of itching and tension in her neck, although she had no pain. The family doctor suggested that Kathy rub a soothing cream into Jessie's neck, but it made little difference. The neck stretching lasted for a couple of months, and then it too gradually disappeared. For a month or so, all was well.

Occasionally, Jessie would make a facial grimace; she called it her funny face. She would roll her eyes or purse her lips. As little movements or habits were now a part of Jessie, Kathy tried to ignore them. The following summer Jessie began to sniff and rub her nose at the same time. Jessie didn't look ill and certainly did not have any signs of a cold or flu. Kathy and Frank were puzzled and consulted the family doctor again. Perhaps Jessie was allergic to something? The doctor prescribed some anti-histamines in case Jessie had an allergy. She took the pills for a month but they made her quite sleepy. The sniffing persisted, so Kathy stopped the tablets. Strangely, Jessie seemed relatively happy and unconcerned about her habits. Her school work progressed and she had friends.

Then something different and more worrying happened. When Jessie went to the supermarket with her mother, she began to touch certain items on the shelves. Her touching rituals became more elaborate. Jessie had to touch things exactly four times and when Kathy asked her why she did so, she simply said, 'I have to'. The touching spread into many other areas—at home, with friends, and even at school. Jessie had always been popular at school, but when she began touching her classmates, their desks, their pens and schoolwork, they naturally began to complain. She also started to arrange things symmetrically. If, for example, her place setting at the dinner table was not perfect, she would spend ages arranging the knife, fork, spoon, glass, and plate until they appeared totally symmetrical to her. She would become excessively concerned with the neatness of her bedroom and all her toys had to have their special places. She became very upset if any of these items were moved. When asked why she did it she cried, 'I can't help it'.

Jessie also began to have bathing and bedtime rituals. She would have to do things a certain number of times and in a certain way. If her routine was interrupted in any way at all, she would have to begin again at the beginning. A bath could quite easily take 30 to 45 minutes. Kathy and Frank were concerned not only that Jessie now seemed unhappy, but that her touching and preoccupation with neatness and symmetry, and her rituals had now become excessive.

Kathy went back to the family doctor who was baffled by the apparent change in Jessie and referred her to a local child psychologist. The psychologist made an assessment and suggested some psychotherapy. Although Jessie liked talking to the psychologist, it made no real difference to her various twitches, nor indeed to her rituals. She was now eleven and the Davis family began to despair.

It was at this point that Kathy read an article in a magazine about a child with Tourette syndrome. There were so many similarities between the child described and Jessie. At the end of the article was the address of the Tourette Syndrome Association. Kathy couldn't wait to tell Frank of her discovery. He agreed that the description of the child's behaviour in the article and that of Jessie was very similar, so Kathy wrote to the Association. Their reply was just what Kathy and Frank needed— some literature on Tourette syndrome and the names and addresses of doctors who specialised in the condition. The family doctor was happy to refer Jessie to a specialist since he himself had been baffled by her symptoms for some time.

The specialist neuropsychiatrist took a careful personal and family history, discovering that Kathy's father cleared his throat repeatedly and that he also had a number of habits. He examined Jessie, reassuring everybody that, as expected, there were no serious abnormalities. He performed tests to rule out other more serious problems and, as expected, they were all normal. Jessie was given medication—a very small dose of haloperidol (Serenace) as well as fluoxetine (Prozac), the latter being in a relatively high dosage. Jessie was also referred to a psychologist specializing in behavioural therapy, to help her learn to deal with all her rituals.

The neuropsychiatrist also reassured the Davis family that Jessie's symptoms would diminish with the treatment, and that she was otherwise a normal well-adjusted child. The only somewhat worrying aspect was that the Tourette syndrome was hereditary—and it appeared to have come from Kathy's side of the family. The prognosis proved to be quite correct. Jessie's symptoms almost disappeared, and she had virtually no side effects from the medication. Jessie was once again a normal, happy child.

Why are these three cases so different?

All three of the individuals described here have Tourette syndrome, but they differ in several ways. In Tim's case it is mild, not causing him distress, and by and large not interfering with his life. Johnny, on the other hand, has Tourette syndrome more severely. His symptoms do interfere with his life and with those around him. Furthermore, Johnny has the accompanying condition of attention deficit hyperactivity disorder (ADHD). Finally, Jessie has moderate Tourette syndrome but with the accompanying condition of obsessive–compulsive behaviour. All three cases are typical, but show different manifestations of the condition. It is not yet known why one person will show mild symptoms whilst another will demonstrate more severe symptoms and may have accompanying problems controlling his or her attention.

2
Questions and answers about Tourette syndrome

How common is Tourette syndrome?

The exact rate depends, at least in part, on how one defines Tourette syndrome, but the generally accepted figure nowadays is five cases per 10 000 people. Using these figures, this would mean there are approximately 110 000 patients in the USA, and 25 000 in the UK. These figures are probably an underestimate. In addition, from large family studies, we have learned that there may be mild cases where a doctor has never been consulted. (Tim's father, described in Chapter 1, is an example of a mild case). Tics are the most common movement disorder in childhood, and it has been estimated that up to 20 percent of school-age children may experience them at some time.

Why is Tourette syndrome diagnosed more frequently these days?

There is an increased awareness of the condition amongst health professionals. Publications in medical literature are frequently followed by radio, TV, and press exposure, and this media attention in turn increases public awareness. In some instances there may even be over-diagnosis by the medical profession. However, worldwide, there are still a large number of individuals who remain undiagnosed.

Does Tourette syndrome occur universally?

Tourette syndrome occurs in all cultures where it has been looked for. Although clinically a rather complex condition, its main characteristics seem to be independent of culture. In other words the symptoms of Tourette syndrome occur with some degree of uniformity irrespective of the country of origin. The majority of studies agree that it is three to four times more common in males than in females. The disorder may be rarer in some ethnic groups eg, Afro-Caribbean. This may be due to either under-recognition, or to genetic factors (which we will discuss later). The disorder is also found in all social classes. Some research suggests that people with Tourette syndrome may be under-achievers.

When does Tourette syndrome begin?

The average age of the onset of symptoms is about seven years old, with the most frequent initial symptoms being excessive eyeblinking or eye-rolling. Patients usually show more complicated movements later. These might include inappropriate licking, smelling, spitting, hitting, jumping, squatting, abnormalities of gait involving posture and movement, and 'forced touching'. The onset of vocal tics usually occurs later than the motor tics, at the average age of 11.

What form do the tics take?

A tic is an abrupt, sudden, jerky repetitive movement or vocalisation which involves discrete muscle groups. They often mimic a normal co-ordinated movement, they vary in intensity and are non-rhythmic. They are experienced as irresistible, but can be suppressed voluntarily for varying lengths of time, often at the expense of inner tension. Both motor and vocal tics may be classified as either simple or complex. Common simple motor tics include eye-blinking, shoulder-shrugging, and facial grimacing. Common complex motor tics include jumping, touching, squatting, licking, or smelling objects. Common simple vocal tics include throat clearing, grunting, sniffing, and snorting. Other complex tics, both motor and vocal, are discussed below.

Coprolalia (the inappropriate and involuntary uttering of obscenities) occurs in about 10 percent of individuals with Tourette syndrome, but may occur in one third of clinic patients. It is rare in children or in mildly affected cases. There is some suggestion that it may be culturally determined, since in one Japanese study it was shown to be rare. If coprolalia occurs at all, it usually begins at around the age of 15.

Copropraxia (the involuntary making of inappropriate obscene gestures), *echolalia* (the imitation of other people's speech), *echopraxia* (imitation of other people's actions), and *palilalia* (the repetition of the patient's own last word, phrase, or syllable) are characteristic symptoms of Tourette syndrome and while they occur not infrequently in clinic populations, their frequency in mild Tourette syndrome individuals is unknown.

Other symptoms, such as *mental coprolalia* (thinking obscene thoughts), *coprographia* (writing obscene words or phrases) and *mental palilalia* (silently saying to oneself the last part of a word heard) become known only when the clinician asks about them directly. These clinical features are not essential to make the diagnosis. (The diagnostic criteria for Tourette syndrome are explained more fully in Chapter 3).

What factors affect tics?

Motor and vocal tics may be aggravated by anxiety, stress, boredom, fatigue, and excitement. In addition, some people have reported that pre-menstrual tension, some food substances (such as additives), and stimulants such as caffeine, methylphenidate, pemoline, and amphetamines, may also make tics worse. In contrast, sleep, alcohol, cannabis, fever, relaxation, playing sport, or concentrating on an enjoyable task may lead to a temporary disappearance of the symptoms.

Do people with Tourette syndrome make socially inappropriate statements?

Patients with Tourette syndrome may demonstrate blurting behaviour. For example, one of us (MR) wears make-up, and most of her clothes have shoulder pads. One patient with Tourette syndrome came up to her during a ward round and, tapping her shoulders (and shoulder pads), said 'Mary Robertson is going to play American football'. Needless to say, there was a laugh, and when things had quietened down he pointed at her again, saying 'Mary Robertson's overdone the blusher!' These personal comments are clearly not the way most people would talk to their doctor. We have another colleague, Dr Walkup, and when he stepped onto the podium to give a lecture, a person with Tourette syndrome shouted, 'Walkup step down!'. People with Tourette syndrome may also make racist or sexist slurs—that is, saying the most inappropriate thing at the time. When this occurs the person with the syndrome is often embarrassed. In many instances, what is blurted out in no way reflects the person's true feelings or beliefs.

Can people with Tourette syndrome also develop other psychiatric conditions?

Several studies have found that clinic patients with Tourette syndrome are more prone to depression than control groups. It has also been suggested that the depression is related to the duration of the condition. This makes good sense, since Tourette syndrome may be a chronic, often socially disabling, and stigmatizing disorder when the symptoms are moderate to severe. Patients with Tourette syndrome are often also more anxious when compared with the general population. We suspect that depression and anxiety are secondary to having Tourette syndrome.

In 1907 Meige and Feindel, in *The confessions of a victim to tic*, described a patient with tics who also had *obsessive–compulsive* behaviour. It is now increasingly evident that there is a strong association between the two conditions, both in patients and in their family members. For example, one study found that patients with Tourette syndrome are disproportionately obsessional, and that this phenomenon is not due to having depression. Other studies have demonstrated differences between pure obsessive–compulsive disorder (OCD) and the apparently similar thoughts and behaviours seen in people with Tourette syndrome. In classic OCD, the majority of *obsessions* (repetitive, senseless, intrusive thoughts) are concerned with worries about dirt, germs or contamination, whilst the majority of *compulsions* (repetitive behaviours) are usually to do with excessive washing. In Tourette syndrome, by contrast, the obsessions are often to do with thoughts about symmetry, counting, and sex and violence, and the compulsions are more concerned with counting, touching, checking, and things being 'just right', and may also involve self injury (see below and also Jessie's case in Chapter 1.) The obsessions and compulsions in Tourette syndrome appear to be independent of the severity of the disorder. Most researchers now believe that some forms of obsessive compulsive behaviour are genetically related to Tourette syndrome.

There also seems to be a link between attention deficit hyperactivity disorder and Tourette syndrome, because ADHD may be common in clinic patients with Tourette syndrome (recall the case of Johnny, in Chapter 1). However, the precise relationship between the two conditions is complex and remains unclear. The characteristic features of ADHD are poor concentration, short attention span, being easily distracted, hyperactivity and impulsiveness. ADHD has been shown to occur in as many as eight percent of boys in the general population. In Tourette syndrome, as many as 50% of patients in some clinics may have some form of ADHD.

Some types of *self injurious behaviour* have also been linked to Tourette syndrome. Even individuals with mild Tourette syndrome may exhibit such behaviours. The types of self-injurious behaviour seem to be similar to those found in people with learning disabilities (mental retardation): e.g. head banging, body-punching, slapping, body-poking, and banging with hard objects. Some of these behaviours may have a compulsive quality to them.

Other behaviours that occur more often than one might expect in clinic patients with Tourette syndrome include antisocial behaviour, including aggression, conduct disorder, and discipline problems. Indeed, these are often the reason for referral in the first place and can be difficult to manage.

There are some clinicians who suggest that a wide variety of psychiatric conditions, such as phobias, alcoholism, drug abuse, gambling, and eating disorders, are highly associated with Tourette syndrome. While some *clinic* patients with severe Tourette syndrome may demonstrate some of these, most people with the syndrome in the community are *not* psychiatrically disturbed in these ways. Finally, in our opinion there is no significant association between Tourette syndrome and psychotic conditions, such as schizophrenia or manic-depressive illness.

Is there more than one type of Tourette syndrome?

There is only one condition known as Tourette syndrome, but because its symptoms are complex, it may be helpful to subdivide it into several categories. At the milder end of the spectrum one may have mild, 'pure' or simple Tourette syndrome, with the motor and vocal tics as the predominant symptoms. Progressing onto a more complex disorder one may have 'full blown' Tourette syndrome, with echophenomena (copying behaviours), palilalia (repeating oneself), coprolalia (swearing tics), copropraxia (obscene gesture tics) and self-injury. Progressing still further one may have Tourette Syndrome 'Plus' in which the individual also has the added problems of obsessive–compulsive behaviour, ADHD, depression and/or anxiety and other psychopathology.

What is St. Vitus's Dance?

Many years ago St. Vitus's dance was diagnosed fairly often. It may have referred to Sydenham's chorea (associated with rheumatic fever) or to Tourette syndrome. Both Sydenham's chorea and Tourette syndrome involve involuntary movements and both are associated with obsessional behaviour. Sydenham's chorea is characterized by choreaform movements. These are random, rapid, fleeting, irregular, dance-like, unpredictable jerks, which are non-repetitive and never integrated into a co-ordinated act. They tend to be aggravated by voluntary movements, stress or anxiety, and disappear during sleep.

What might be wrong at the psychological level?

Most people with Tourette syndrome have been assessed as having normal intelligence, although on IQ tests their non-verbal abilities may be as much as 15 points lower than their verbal abilities. Some sufferers also have specific difficulties in reading, writing, and arithmetic. These may be the result of disrupted schooling, contributing to their academic underachievement. A recent study has suggested that the *intention editor* is poorly developed in children with Tourette syndrome. The intention editor is a mechanism thought to underlie action control and begins to function in early childhood. It is normally triggered whenever there are several intentions competing in parallel with each other, such as when you should refrain from saying one thing, whilst saying something else. It may be part of what psychologists also call 'executive function' or 'executive control'.

Finally, some studies have reported difficulties in attention, especially on more complex tasks such as choice reaction time, timed continuous performance tasks, serial addition (keeping a running total in your head), block sequence span (keeping track of the order of doing things), the trail making test (keeping track of a route) and letter cancellation tasks (keeping track of key items). If a child with Tourette syndrome also has ADHD, they may be even more disadvantaged from an educational point of view. If an individual has obsessive–compulsive behaviour, he or she may be very slow and pedantic in the ways in which they do things and think, and this may also leave them disadvantaged.

Is there a biochemical cause of Tourette syndrome?

The neurochemical basis for Tourette syndrome is, as yet, unknown. However, the main biochemical theory is that there is an imbalance in the function of neurotransmitter (a messenger in the brain) called *dopamine*. This theory is based mainly on the beneficial effect of dopamine-blocking drugs, and on the fact that certain stimulants, such as pemoline and methylphenidate, can cause tics to worsen.

However, a number of studies have found other neurochemical abnormalities. For example, patients with Tourette syndrome seem to have lower levels of *serotonin*, another neurotransmitter which concentrates in areas of the brain called the subthalamus and the basal ganglia. There also seems to be a reduction in cyclic AMP (another chemical messenger in the brain). Other abnormalities that have been found include alterations in the noradrenergic system, and an increased number of dopamine uptake carrier sites in the striatum of the brain. In a few cases a decrease in dynorphin (a naturally-occurring opioid-like substance) has been demonstrated in the globus pallidus (part of the basal ganglia). Finally, abnormalities of the opoid system have been found in the frontal areas of the brain. All of these brain areas are shown in Figures 2 and 3.

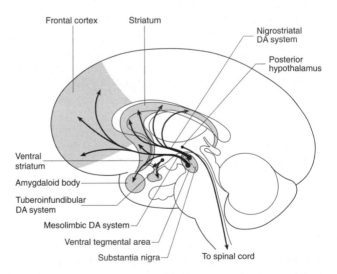

Figure 2 The dopamine pathways in the brain. From L. Heimer (1983). *The human brain and spinal cord.* Springer Verlag, New York.

Have researchers been able to pinpoint the affected areas of the brain?

So far there have been very few post-mortem studies of the brain tissues of people with Tourette syndrome. Those that have been reported show abnormalities in the basal ganglia (an area of the brain concerned with movement) and the anterior cingulate cortex, and their connections with the periaqueductal grey matter and midbrain tegmentum (see Figures 2 and 3).

Does electrophysiology reveal any abnormalities?

Electroencephalographic (EEG) testing measures electrical activity in the brain. Studies show that in patients with Tourette syndrome EEG patterns are mostly normal, but if abnormalities are found they are minor and non-specific. There is also no specific relationship between epilepsy and Tourette syndrome.

What does neuroimaging (brain scanning) reveal?

Neuroimaging has revolutionized the way we study the brain, but in Tourette syndrome, these techniques are used mainly in research, rather than in routine clinical practice. They reveal two aspects of the brain:

1. Structure of the brain

Computerized tomography (CT) scans of the brain have not revealed any abnormalities that might throw light on the cause of Tourette syndrome. There have been a few cases of abnormal CT scans documented in the medical literature, but by far the majority have been normal. Magnetic resonance imaging (MRI) scans of the structure of the brain have been able to detect more subtle abnormalities than have CT scans. Fairly consistent abnormalities which have been reported include abnormalities of the caudate nucleus size (the caudate nucleus is part of the basal ganglia), the size of the corpus callosum (which divides and transfers information across the two halves of the brain), the symmetry of other basal ganglia, the size of the lateral ventricles, and loss of normal ventricular asymmetry (see Figure 3).

2. Functioning in the brain

Functional imaging of the brain using positron emission tomography (PET) has found metabolic and blood flow abnormalities in the basal ganglia, as well as the fronto-temporal areas, especially in the putamen (see Figures 2 and 3). Studies examining cerebral blood flow using single photon emission computerized tomography (SPET) have again found lower levels of blood flow in the basal ganglia, thalamus and frontal and temporal cortical areas, as well as elevated frontal cortex blood flow (relative to the basal ganglia, and again including the caudate nucleus and putamen).

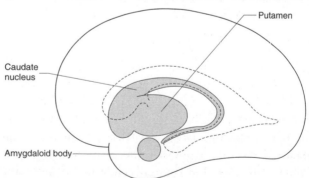

Figure 3 The candate and putamen viewed from the side of the brain. From L. Heimer (1983). *The human brain and spinal cord.* Springer Verlag, New York.

In summary, it seems that both functional and subtle structural abnormalities are found in the brains of people with Tourette syndrome, especially in the fronto-temporal areas and the basal ganglia.

Are genetic factors involved in causing Tourette syndrome?

There is no doubt that genetic factors are involved in Tourette syndrome in the majority of cases, but the precise mechanisms of inheritance are unknown. A few sporadic cases of Tourette syndrome do occur and these must be due to acquired abnormalities in the brain, such as in the basal ganglia.

To date, the genetic basis of Tourette syndrome has not been discovered and there is no blood test for the disorder. We will therefore discuss some of the main genetic hypotheses advanced so far.

Four ways in which Tourette syndrome might be passed down have been suggested. These genetic models are:

(1) autosomal dominant
(2) mixed model
(3) polygenic model
(4) bilinear inheritance.

Most support to date has been for *autosomal dominant* inheritance. This means that, if an individual has Tourette syndrome, there is a 50–50 chance that each offspring will inherit the gene. However, there is a suggestion of *incomplete penetrance*. This means that even if one has the gene, it is not 100 percent the case that the individual will display the symptoms. This type of inheritance suggests the presence of *one single major gene*. It has also been suggested that obsessive–compulsive behaviour may be one of the symptoms (or part of the phenotype) caused by the gene. That is, if an individual inherits the gene, he or she might display obsessive–compulsive behaviour instead of, or as well as, Tourette syndrome.

The second model—the *mixed model*—suggests one major gene but which does not behave strictly according to classic (Mendelian) laws: it is intermediate between recessive (requiring two genes) and dominant (only requiring one gene to be manifest). In this model it is suggested that there is a genetic predisposition involving one copy of the gene which renders an individual vulnerable, and other factors (such as infections, or factors in pregnancy or at birth) determine the extent of the expression of the gene. The number of genes (one or two) may in turn determine the severity of the disorder in any given individual.

A third model—the *polygenic model*—is, to date, somewhat controversial. In this model, multiple genes are involved and no single gene exerts a major effect. In this model it is proposed that there is a threshold number of several genes required to produce Tourette syndrome within a given individual.

The fourth pattern of inheritance which has been described is *bilineality*—that is, an individual inherits the genetic vulnerability from both the maternal and paternal sides.

To complicate matters yet further, it has recently been suggested that there may be *genetic heterogeneity*—ie, different genes may be responsible for Tourette syndrome in different families.

The majority of chromosomes in patients with Tourette syndrome are normal. Chromosomes are composed of genes which are blueprints for making proteins which are the building blocks of life. The search for the Tourette syndrome gene(s) is currently taking place around the world. There is also an international research consortium of nine centres investigating the genetic cause of Tourette syndrome.

To date, no genetic linkage studies have been replicated and much of the genome has been excluded—that is, no particular gene has yet been found to be the cause of Tourette syndrome. In addition many authorities believe that an individual may inherit a vulnerability to a spectrum disorder, including Tourette syndrome, obsessive–compulsive behaviours, and possibly ADHD.

Do other factors besides inheritance cause Tourette syndrome?

A number of factors may be important in determining just how the symptoms of Tourette syndrome are expressed. Perinatal (around birth) factors may interact with genetic factors to cause Tourette syndrome. There have been some recent studies suggesting that the body's autoimmune mechanisms may play a role in the onset or exacerbation of Tourette or obsessive symptoms.

Which therapies are most useful for patients with Tourette syndrome?

Both counselling and medication have proved useful in treating people with Tourette syndrome. For many adult patients with a mild form of the condition, explanation and reassurance may be sufficient. Similarly, parents of mildly affected children may feel that the diagnosis and an explanation about the nature of

Tourette syndrome, plus information about self-help groups, and booklets for teachers, are sufficient. For severely affected patients, who may have the associated features of obsessive–compulsive behaviour, attention deficit and hyperactivity disorder (ADHD), self-injury or aggressive behaviour, the management is more complex.

Individual psychotherapy is useful for reducing and coping with the daily difficulties of living with tics, but the tics themselves are not responsive to psychotherapy and should therefore not be the target of treatment.

Behaviour therapies have been used in Tourette syndrome, including for example: (i) massed negative practice; (ii) relaxation training; and (iii) contingency management. The technique most frequently used has been *massed negative practice* (over-rehearsal of the target tic; such as excessive blinking) in which the patient performs the movement for a specified time, interspersed with periods of rest: it is suggested to the patient that he becomes tired of doing the tic, resulting in a decrease in its frequency. This method does show some therapeutic benefit in Tourette syndrome.

Contingency management holds that behaviours are maintained by the consequences that follow them. Therefore, patients are positively reinforced (using, for example, praise) for not performing tics or performing alternative behaviours. This has been used mainly on children with some success. This method is usually used in combination with other behavioural methods.

Relaxation training has also been used in combination with other methods and includes, for example, muscular tensing and relaxing and deep breathing—

and this may help to reduce the tics for a short period of time.

In summary, behaviour therapy plays a role in the effective management of Tourette syndrome especially in patients with a simple motor or vocal tic and obsessive–compulsive behaviour. It may be useful as an adjunct to medication, or when used alone in patients who are not responding to any treatments, or who experience unwanted side-effects of medication.

Which medications are recommended?

To date there is no cure for Tourette syndrome but there are many medications which successfully reduce the various manifestations.

Medication is, at present, the main treatment for the motor and vocal tics, as well as some of the associated behaviours. The medications most commonly used are the neuroleptics, antipsychotics or dopamine antagonists (such as haloperidol, pimozide, sulpiride, tiapride, and risperidone). These medications are also called major tranquillizers, not because they tranquillize people (especially not people with Tourette syndrome, as they are given relatively small doses), but as a way of differentiating them from the minor tranquillizers or anxiolytics (mainly the diazepam/valium family of drugs). Another reason for the distinction is that, in higher doses, the neuroleptics are administered for traditionally major psychiatric illnesses (such as mania or schizophrenia), whereas the anxiolytics are given for traditionally relatively minor ailments (such as anxiety and sleep disturbances).

Clonidine (often also used in the treatment of

headaches, migraine, and hypertension or high blood pressure) has also been used with some success to reduce the tics in Tourette syndrome. It is especially recommended if a child has Tourette syndrome and associated ADHD. Clonidine can also be taken as a transdermal patch on the skin. Recently Guanfaline has also been shown to be useful and may well have less side effects than Clonidine. Other medications for the ADHD aspects include methylphenidate and pemoline, as well as desipramine and imipramine.

Finally the relatively new specific serotonin reuptake inhibitors (SSRIs) (eg, fluoxetine, fluvoxamine, sertraline, paroxetine, citalopram) can be used to treat the obsessive–compulsive behaviour aspects of the syndrome, as well as when the patient is depressed. SSRIs can also be helpful with impulse control difficulties. The doses, however are different, being higher (eg, fluoxetine 60 mgm daily) for obsessive–compulsive aspects of Tourette syndrome, and lower (eg fluoxetine 20 mgm daily) for depression.

The older tricyclic antidepressant clomipramine, which also acts on serotonin, is useful for the obsessive–compulsive aspects and depression. The many side-effects of clomipramine and the fact that it is dangerous in overdose, make it less acceptable to some. Recently Tetrabenazine has also been documented as useful in reducing symptoms of Tourette Syndrome.

Newer pharmacological strategies have been tried with some success, but to date only with relatively small numbers of patients. These include nicotine transdermal patches (worn on the skin), calcium channel blockers and injections of botulinum toxin into localized areas (e.g. for excessive eye blinking, also known as blepharospasm).

What are the side-effects of these medications?

Side-effects (such as dystonia (stiffness), rigidity, and tremor), as well as sedation and depression are common with haloperidol, but are less so with pimozide. The neuroleptics may also cause concentration problems, cognitive blunting and, rarely, tardive dyskinesia (a movement disorder that consists of lip, mouth, and tongue movements). Sulpiride has fewer side-effects of this sort (that is, fewer extrapyramidal problems) as well as fewer sedative side-effects, although gyneacomastia (enlargement of the breasts in men), galactorrhoea (excessive, unnatural production of milk by the breasts), menstrual irregularities, and depression have been reported.

With the neuroleptics, these side-effects can be avoided by starting with small doses (eg a haloperidol dose of 0.5 mg daily) and increasing the dose by 0.5 mg every week until a point is reached with maximal benefit and minimal side-effect. Reports about changes in electrocardiogram (heart beat) patterns with pimozide have, naturally, raised some concern, so it is important that patients have a baseline electrocardiogram (ECG) to rule out any heart problems. If the patient has the heart condition called the long QT Syndrome, pimozide should not be used. If there are other heart problems, the patient should have routine ECGs under the guidance of a cardiologist. Prescribing neuroleptics to children with Tourette's Syndrome may also be useful, but again there are reports of side-effects which therefore require careful monitoring.

Clonidine has fewer and milder side-effects than the neuroleptics in general, the most common being sedation. This sedation occurs in around 10–20 percent of cases, is dose-related, and with time tolerance often develops. Other side-effects include insomnia, nocturnal restlessness, dry mouth, headaches, dizziness, postural hypotension (lowering of blood pressure especially when standing up) and, occasionally, rashes. The tricyclics can cause dry mouth, constipation, blurring of vision and dizziness. The SSRIs can cause gastric upset, such as nausea. Methylphenidate and pemoline, which are stimulants, can cause loss of appetite and weight, initial insomnia (difficulty in falling asleep), gastrointestinal upset (eg, nausea), and headaches.

Tetrabenazine has also been used with success in Tourette syndrome. It reduces presynaptic (before the nerve ending) monoamines, and blocks postsynaptic (after the nerve ending) dopamine receptors. The main advantage of tetrabenazine is that it rarely causes side-effects such as dystonia (acute stiffness) or tardive dyskinesia (mouth movements after long term high dosage standard neuroleptics). Side-effects which do occur include drowsiness, fatigue, depression, difficulty with sleep, and a feeling of foot/leg restlessness.

Can allergies cause Tourette syndrome?

It has been reported that tics can worsen with seasonal allergies, or when allergens in food are eaten. Also drugs used to treat allergies may increase tics. Although there may be food intolerance in some patients, to date there is little scientific evidence of the involvement of allergy in Tourette syndrome. Individual patients may be allergic to certain substances (eg, chocolate) and they are of course advised to avoid these foods. People with Tourette syndrome are affected by allergies in no greater number than the general population.

What is the typical outcome for a child with Tourette syndrome?

Tourette syndrome is usually lifelong. This was most dramatically illustrated by the case of the Marquise de Dampierre, who was originally seen by Itard in 1825, and who apparently continued to show tics until she was elderly. As mentioned earlier, across a person's life, new tics may appear and older ones disappear. During adolescence the symptoms tend to reach a peak and to be more unpredictable from day to day. They may then begin to subside.

It has also been shown that up to nearly three quarters of patients report that their tics decrease markedly or even disappear during the latter years of adolescence or early adulthood. However, along with this reduction of tics after early adulthood, there may not be an improvement in the associated behavioural difficulties. In addition, some patients may even experience an increase in these during late adulthood, even if there has been a remission. Stress in later life, such as divorce or a death in the family, can also cause a re-emergence of tics.

To the best of our knowledge one of the predictors of outcome is the severity of symptoms at the end of adolescence. However, the severity of the tics is not the only factor which predicts an individual's long-term adjustment and outcome; the associated behaviours and emotional problems of adjustment are also important. In addition, poor prognosis are associated with trauma, mental retardation (learning disability), obsessive–compulsive features, and attention deficit disorder.

Have any famous people had Tourette syndrome?

Dr Oliver Sacks has helped publicize Tourette syndrome for many years. In his books *The Man Who Mistook his Wife for a Hat* and *An Anthropologist on Mars*, he has given wide and sympathetic coverage to people with Tourette syndrome. Dr Sacks describes 'phantasmagoric Touretters' who seem almost super-human, with exceptional creativity, charisma, sense of humour, and productive energy. A play based on Oliver Sacks' book, called *The Man Who* was directed by Peter Brooke in London and Paris, and helped portray Tourette syndrome to theatre audiences (see Figure 4).

However, most people with the syndrome are not exceptional. Those who have mild Tourette syndrome (the majority) live quite unnoticed in their communities, pursuing their daily business in all walks of life. People who have severe Tourette syndrome may be socially disadvantaged, with few friends, have unemployment as a constant burden, and experience sadness about the stigmatization attached to having a so-called bizarre disorder.

We know of several famous people who are thought to have had Tourette syndrome. Without doubt the most accomplished is Dr Samuel Johnson, the English literary giant who also appears to have had associated obsessive–compulsive behaviour, echophenomena, mild self-injurious behaviour and depression (see Figure 5). Others include Tolstoy's brother Dmitry (described in the novel *Anna Karenina* and portrayed in the character Nicolai Levin), Julius Wechter (the marimba player of the 1960s group, Herb Alpert's Tijuana Brass), and the American major league baseball hero, Jim Eisenreich.

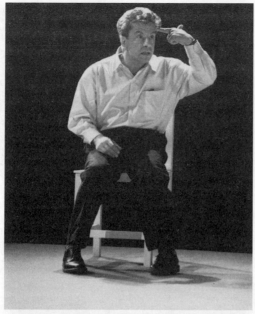

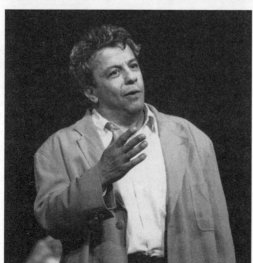

Figure 4 Maurice Benichou in '*l'homme qui*' ('The Man Who'), Centre International de Creations Théâtrales, Paris. Photograph courtesy of Gilles Abegg.

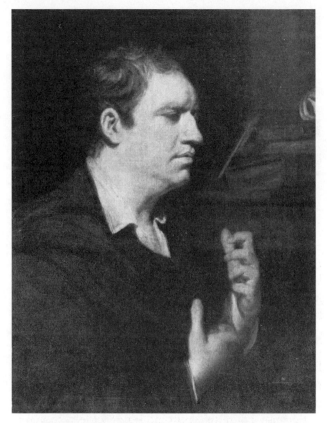

Figure 5 Samuel Johnson in 1770, painted by Joshua Reynolds. Reproduced from John Wain (1974) *Samuel Johnson*, MacMillan Ltd, London.

In the next chapter, we describe in detail how the diagnosis of Tourette syndrome is made.

3
How the diagnosis is made

A diagnosis is essential if different conditions are to be clearly distinguished from one another and is important in the understanding and treatment of such conditions. In the case of Tourette syndrome, early diagnosis offers the hope that management can begin before the syndrome pushes the individual too far off the normal course of development, resulting in problems with education, relationships, and career.

Because Tourette syndrome is not widely known it may go unrecognized. Indeed many patients are diagnosed only when they reach adolescence or adulthood. It is hoped that with better education of both professionals and the lay public, earlier recognition and thus earlier diagnosis will take place. However, despite having heard of Tourette syndrome, some doctors are unwilling to make a firm diagnosis. Others still labour under the misapprehension that coprolalia (involuntary inappropriate swearing) must be present for the diagnosis of Tourette syndrome to be made.

Tourette syndrome was once thought to be rare but now it is being recognized and diagnosed increasingly often. In this chapter we describe an assessment format used at the National Hospital for Neurology and Neurosurgery in London. This format is basically similar to diagnostic methods used in other countries where there are specialists in Tourette syndrome. We also clarify how Tourette syndrome can be distinguished from superficially similar conditions. Finally, we discuss the implications and consequences of receiving a confirmed diagnosis.

How patients are referred to the clinic

Often parents bring their child to the clinic after having been referred by their family doctor. Initially, the parents themselves suspect the child has symptoms of the condition. Their suspicions may have been aroused by seeing a television programme, or reading an article about someone with Tourette syndrome. In many countries family doctors or parents find specialist clinics through a local or national Tourette Syndrome Association (see Appendix 3) which keeps a list of doctors who are familiar with diagnosing and treating patients with the syndrome.

The diagnosis

Tourette syndrome is a *syndrome* (a disorder in which there is a clustering of a number of essential characteristic symptoms, which may include a number of other characteristic features and associated behaviours).

Motor and vocal tics

The essential features of Tourette syndrome are the presence of multiple motor tics (twitches) and one or more vocal tics (or noises). The tics may appear simultaneously or at different times throughout the illness. Typically the tics occur many times a day, in bouts, and must have been present for at least one year if a diagnosis is to be made. The doctor making the diagnosis will also check the age of symptom onset of Tourette syndrome, because this is usually before the age of 18.

The doctor will ask about the anatomical location (ie, which part of the body) the tics are in, and the number, frequency, complexity, and severity of the tics as they change over time. The motor tics may involve the following areas of the body:

- head and face: (eg, excessive eye-blinking or squinting, eye-rolling, nose twitches, mouth opening, tongue protrusion, making faces, nodding or turning of the head sideways)
- shoulders (shrugging)
- arms (jerking)
- legs (kicking)
- abdominal contractions (tummy pulling in).

Complex tics include smelling and licking things, spitting, touching of parts of the body, forced touching of objects, abnormalities of gait (such as funny walking, twirling), squatting, hopping, skipping, and bending down.

Simple vocal tics include sounds such as repetitive sniffing, snorting, throat clearing, coughing, and gulping. *Complex vocal tics* include whistling and belching. Animal noises similar to a dog yelping or barking, duck, and pig noises can also occur.

Other characteristic features

Concern need not be felt if the doctor asks about coprolalia (the inappropriate, involuntary, and often disguised uttering of obscenities and blasphemous words), since this must be checked. It occurs in about 10 percent of individuals with Tourette syndrome. The full word need not be uttered and so the doctor may ask if the patient says merely 'fu' or disguises the word and says 'fick', followed by a cough and covering of the mouth. Copropraxia (the inappropriate, involuntary and often disguised making of obscene gestures such as the 'V' sign or 'third finger' sign) occurs in a few patients, so again this will be enquired about specifically.

Next there are another set of symptoms which will be specifically checked. Does the patient demonstrate any of the following:

- echolalia (copying what other people say, eg repeating what they say or copying their accents)
- echopraxia (copying what other people do, eg copying their movements)
- palilalia (repeating oneself over and over, especially the last word or phrase said)
- palipraxia (repetitive movements eg repeatedly doing up a button over and over again)

These symptoms occur in a substantial proportion of people with Tourette syndrome, but often have to be specifically enquired after. Not all symptoms occur in all patients.

Associated features and disorders

As mentioned in Chapter 2, the most characteristic associated symptoms are obsessions and compulsions. *Obsessions* are persistent ideas, thoughts, impulses or images which are experienced as intrusive, inappropriate, senseless and repetitive. *Compulsions* are repetitive behaviours (eg hand-washing, ordering, checking) which are performed in order to prevent or reduce anxiety or distress.

Because obsessions and compulsions are disturbing for the patient, they are technically called 'egodystonic' (unwanted and intrusive). As mentioned in Chapter 2, in obsessive–compulsive disorder (OCD), the common obsessions often have to do with dirt, germs, and contamination. The resultant compulsions have to do with cleaning and washing. Obsessional doubting, and therefore repetitive checking, are also common. However, in Tourette syndrome, the obsessions often involve thinking about violent scenes, sexual thoughts, and counting (arithmomania), and the compulsions have to do with symmetry, 'evening up', lining things up and getting things 'just right'. To contrast it with OCD, many people refer to these behaviours in Tourette syndrome as obsessive–compulsive behaviours (OCB). If the doctor asks about these things, it is to check if the diagnosis should be of 'pure' Tourette syndrome, or Tourette syndrome with obsessive–compulsive behaviours, or even OCD.

Attention deficit hyperactivity disorder (ADHD) is characterized by poor concentration and attention, being easily distracted, impulsiveness, and hyperactivity. It is relatively common in people with Tourette syndrome, especially children, where ADHD may often cause disruption in the school classroom and cause difficulties with education for the child and his or her classmates. The doctor will again need to check if the appropriate diagnosis is 'pure' Tourette syndrome, or Tourette syndrome with ADHD.

Other distressing associated behaviours include self-injury (such as head banging or body punching), which can be dangerous. Depression is also quite common in clinic patients with Tourette syndrome. Any of these associated behaviours will be noted because they will obviously have implications for management and treatment.

It is, nevertheless, important to realize that many people with Tourette syndrome are only mildly affected, live in the community, never seek medical attention, and may not be distressed by their symptoms.

The assessment

Although there are a number of different approaches to assessing individuals with Tourette syndrome, the basic principles are usually the same at different centres.

In the first place, a thorough *history* must be taken, enquiring specifically about the occurrence of tics, their progression, enquiring about other characteristic symptoms, and also about the associated behaviours. In some clinics, specialized *interview schedules* are used to gather the information in a standardized way so as to make an accurate diagnosis, to be sure of enquiring about all the associated features, and to enable the clinician to make an accurate assessment of the severity of the symptoms. The history is usually taken from both the patient and another informant (eg a parent, carer, spouse, or teacher).

The clinician has to perform a *neurological assessment* (examining the nerves and the muscle reflexes) because there are sometimes subtle abnormalities in Tourette syndrome and other neurological disorders need to be excluded. The clinician will then also perform a *mental state examination* to look for depression (which can occur in Tourette syndrome) and to exclude other psychiatric conditions, such as psychosis (eg schizophrenia or mania). This takes the form of some standard questioning. It is important to exclude schizophrenia and mania as they can be treated, but it is not common to find them in association with Tourette syndrome.

Special investigations may be recommended, such as *blood tests* to exclude Wilson's disease (an abnormality of copper). Usually no further tests are undertaken, but if there are atypical features, the clinician may refer the person for one or more of the following tests: an *electroencephalogram* (EEG), which is a harmless investigation involving fixing small discs to the scalp and recording the activity of the brain; or a *brain scan* which may involve computerized tomography (CT) or magnetic resonance imaging (MRI). Positron emission tomography (PET) or single photon emission computed tomography (SPECT) are usually performed for research purposes. These were all mentioned in Chapter 2 in detail. Such scans are undertaken to exclude other less common causes of tics, or abnormalities such as epilepsy.

Neuropsychological testing (often involving IQ or intelligence testing) may also show differences in the child's verbal and non-verbal IQ, even if the child's overall IQ is in the normal range.

An electrocardiogram (ECG, a test recording the activity of the heart) must be performed if certain drugs (eg pimozide) are to be prescribed, as abnormalities of the ECG can occur with pimozide.

Clinicians experienced in assessing and managing patients with Tourette syndrome are usually able to do this whole evaluation on an out-patient basis, when the assessment can last between two and four hours. Often a lunch break will be included, since these tests can be tiring for the family and the patient. If the problems are complex or difficult, a period of in-patient assessment may occasionally be required.

It is ideal for clinics to be multidiscipliniary and include a psychiatrist, neurologist, clinical psychologist, behaviour therapist, social worker, and an educational psychologist. However, this may well be too expensive for hospitals in the public sector. Sadly, many clinics are staffed by a minimum of professionals.

In our clinic in London we routinely provide the patient and their family with a personalized Fact Sheet, explaining which symptoms they have, the medical names for the symptoms, the severity of their Tourette syndrome and the associated behaviours. We also include current information about the causes and treatment of Tourette syndrome.

Local and national self-help groups

After giving a diagnosis of Tourette syndrome, in many clinics, if the patient and their family are unaware of the local or national Tourette Syndrome Association (TSA) (see Appendix 3), it is common for the doctor to put them in touch with it. In some countries, a 'Questions and Answers' leaflet from the Association is available, which includes basic information about Tourette syndrome. These leaflets are routinely handed out in our clinic after the diagnosis.

The TSAs usually provide additional advice, details about local support groups, and information regarding recent developments in treatment and research. For the child, specific treatments (see Chapter 2) and educational provisions (see Chapter 4) may be arranged, depending on the nature of the problems and the age of the child. The various TSAs also hold regular meetings for patients, their relatives, and interested professionals.

Distinguishing Tourette syndrome from other conditions

The task for the clinician is to decide whether the patient has Tourette's syndrome or some other similar condition. Sometimes he has to decide whether both Tourette syndrome and another condition are present.

Tourette syndrome can be confused with a number of other conditions. It may, for example, appear similar to any of the following:

- *transient tic disorder* (TTD, in which single or multiple motor and or vocal tics occur for at least four weeks, but do not last longer than 12 consecutive months);
- *chronic motor or vocal tic disorder* (in which single or multiple motor *or* vocal tics, *but not both,* last for longer than a year);
- *Sydenham's Chorea* (St Vitus's dance, a movement disorder which occurs more frequently in females, usually children, and 75 per cent of cases are associated with rheumatic fever);
- *Huntington's disease* (a movement disorder which usually begins between the ages of 30 and 50, but may occur in childhood and which is associated with early behavioural problems and later dementia. There is usually a family history of Huntington's chorea);
- *Tardive Tourettism*, a syndrome following treatment with neuroleptics (eg haloperidol, or pimozide);

- *dystonia* (twisting of certain muscle groups, often the legs, which is usually crippling and progressive);
- *spasmodic torticollis* (involving a wry neck, which usually begins between the ages of 30 and 50 years);
- *Wilson's disease* (usually presenting between the ages of 10 and 25 years, with characteristic signs in the eye and liver, and with abnormal copper in the blood and urine);
- *epilepsy* (when the patient may have seizures or fits during which they have jerking movements, usually associated with a loss of consciousness);
- *myoclonic epilepsy* (a type of epilepsy in which there is muscle jerking with no loss of consciousness).

Table 1 Conditions not to be confused with Tourette syndrome

Transient tic disorder
Chronic multiple tic disorder
Sydenham's chorea
Huntington's disease
Tardive tourettism
Dystonia
Spasmodic torticollis
Wilson's disease
Epilepsy
Myoclonic epilepsy
Autism
Learning disability

Finally, some children with *autism* (a condition primarily involving abnormalities of social interaction, peer relationships, language, communication, together with restricted, repetitive patterns of behaviour) may have echolalia, abnormal postures, and obsessive–compulsive type of behaviours. In such cases, this might simply resemble Tourette syndrome, or Tourette syndrome and autism might actually co-occur. Some individuals with learning disability (also called mental handicap) have this and stereotyped behaviours. This set of conditions with which Tourette syndrome should not be confused is summarized in Table 1.

Other conditions and behavioural problems

We have already mentioned that a proportion of children and adults with Tourette syndrome have a history of childhood ADHD and OCB. Quite often it is these behaviours, and not the motor and vocal tics *per se*, which are a matter of concern and warrant treatment.

In addition, some children and many adults with Tourette syndrome who attend clinics have symptoms of *depression* which also requires appropriate recognition and treatment in its own right. Children may also have *conduct disorder* and, once again, it is this which may be the cause for concern, rather than the motor and vocal tics.

Typical signs of conduct disorder include bullying, threatening or intimidating others, starting physical fights, using a harmful weapon, physical cruelty to people and animals, repetitive stealing and lying, destroying others' property, fire-setting, staying out at night, running away from home, and playing truant. Some children with conduct disorder grow up into adults with a *personality disorder* (eg antisocial behaviours such as stealing and aggression). It is these behaviours which may cause more problems than do the motor or vocal tics. There is no specific medication prescribed for individuals with conduct and personality disorders. Firm (though kind) handling is required to try and encourage them to conform to the social norms of society, and to make them aware of the consequences of not adhering to them.

In our experience, the majority of individuals in the community with Tourette syndrome do not have these problems, although patients in the *clinic* may. This over-representation of people with problems in specialist clinics is called referral bias.

Immediate consequences of diagnosis

If you or your child's condition fits the clinical picture of Tourette syndrome, at first it may seem that your worst fears have come true. Secretly you may have been hoping to hear that the problems were only mild and would pass. The diagnosis may then be a shock. There are, however, many different reactions and many different stages in the reaction to the diagnosis of Tourette syndrome.

Many of the children who are diagnosed are unaware of the implications of diagnosis and are thus largely unaffected by receiving it. Parents and adult patients differ widely in their reactions to the diagnosis.

Whatever the response, parents and patients often feel apprehension about the future and confusion about the condition. Receipt of a confirmed Tourette syndrome diagnosis should be followed up by sensitive discussion with the family (parents, spouse, partner) about the nature of the problems, their severity, and the expected future course. Further information and support should always be provided.

Why is Tourette syndrome not diagnosed in infancy?

As we mentioned earlier, Tourette syndrome usually becomes evident at around the age of seven, with the onset of the motor tics. However, some children do begin with hyperactivity or obsessive–compulsive behaviour. The question then arises, why is Tourette syndrome not picked up in infancy? At present it is rare to diagnose the condition before the age of five or so, and in many instances it is not diagnosed until considerably later.

There are a number of reasons for this delay. First, before the ages of five to seven years, the patterns of behaviour and history of motor and vocal tics may not be clear enough to allow a definitive diagnosis to be made. Secondly, children with Tourette syndrome may also have ADHD and it may be that the ADHD is the main cause for concern, and a focus on this may mean that the Tourette syndrome goes undetected. Thirdly, in most children with Tourette syndrome, there is a period of normal development and only later do the motor and vocal tics and associated behaviours develop. Fourthly, because of the tendency of tics to wax and wane and change over time, it may take some time for the doctor to obtain a complete picture of the symptoms. Finally, because children (and adults) often suppress their symptoms in the company of strangers, including doctors, the tics may not be seen or heard and the diagnosis therefore not made.

There is as yet no blood test which can be taken from the mother in pregnancy, nor from the child, which can confirm the diagnosis of Tourette syndrome. This contrasts with procedure in disorders where a gene has been identified, and blood tests can confirm a diagnosis (eg Huntington's disease). Therefore this also means that prenatal detection of Tourette syndrome is not yet possible.

In addition to these reasons, a late diagnosis may occur simply because parents (or adult patients) have little experience of the development and behaviour of normal children, hence they may be unaware of the problems in their or their child's behaviour. Tim the teacher's case (in Chapter 1) was just such an example. 'All children have the odd tic, don't they?' is a common statement we have heard. After all, no parents like to think that their child has a problem. The GP or health visitor may also have difficulties identifying subtle symptoms of Tourette syndrome (eg mild tics), and instead feel that they are simply transient developmental problems. This is not very surprising, given that it is unlikely for one of these health professionals to see even a single case of diagnosed Tourette syndrome during their whole career. As a consequence, parents are often told, 'He'll grow out of it'. As mentioned earlier, it is hoped that, in time, primary health professionals will become better able to detect possible cases of Tourette syndrome and refer such cases on to specialists at younger ages, for suitable early intervention.

4
Coping with the news

To discover your child has a condition which may result in potential lifelong disability is, naturally, a tremendous blow. When parents finally realize that their child has Tourette syndrome, and that it is not 'just a difficult phase he's going through', they may feel like they have 'lost' the 'wonderful and normal' child they thought they had and they may be overwhelmed by a wide range of emotions: sometimes despair and depression, as well as anxiety about their child's future.

At times a cloak of guilt can envelop them, making them feel in some way responsible for their child's condition. 'Was it in my genes?', 'Was it bad parenting?'. On occasion, they may feel a pervasive sense of shame or embarrassment, due to the perceived opinions of others: 'They've failed as parents—listen to their child swearing!—and he's so young.' Whilst noticing the child is swearing is an accurate observation, it does not mean they have failed as parents, of course, since the child's condition is no one's fault. All of these emotions are understandable reactions to the stresses and disappointments induced by the child's developmental problems, tics, noises, and at times erratic behaviour. When adults receive a diagnosis there may also be a variety of conflicting emotions. There may be anger, with the obvious question, 'Why me? Why us?'.

Emotional reactions following the discovery of disabling conditions

A fair amount is known about how parents respond to the discovery that their child has a disability. The following account is a description of the type of feelings that immediately follow when parents are told that their child has a medical condition like autism, Down syndrome, epilepsy, or cystic fibrosis. We begin with this description because it best illustrates the range of feelings and thoughts that can occur in these circumstances. However, since Tourette syndrome is also very different from all these other conditions, this description is followed by an outline of how the reaction to the discovery of Tourette syndrome may be different.

Not surprisingly, the immediate reactions are sometimes similar to those seen following bereavement: an initial phase of shock and disbelief (parents sometimes talk of feeling numb or cut off from the world). To some extent, the numbness helps prevent parents from being overwhelmed by their distress, and seems to act as a means of buffering them from the full significance of the discovery.

Understandably, parents find it difficult to assimilate new information during this period, and they may need to go through things several times at a later stage to grasp them fully. As a consequence, doctors should try to keep information short and simple when initially discussing the diagnosis, and then go through the details when parents have had a chance to recover from hearing the news. As described already, we routinely hand out a very simple Fact Sheet so that parents or patients can take it home, absorb the facts, and at their next appointment, ask relevant questions.

The early shock may be followed by a period of denial. Denial may be the mind's way of keeping anxiety and stress at bay. In its most pronounced form, it may result in people acting as if nothing has occurred: but usually it leads to parents minimizing the seriousness of the conditions and fantasizing that their child will somehow be magically 'cured' or grow out of it.

The next phase of the reaction is often full of feelings of anger and guilt. Anger at the injustice of the tragedy ('How could this happen to me?' 'What have I done to deserve this?' 'Why my child?'), and guilt ('What did we do as parents to cause this?) turning to sadness and despair ('How can we ever cope?'). Finally, most parents adapt and become able to form a realistic picture of the problems, as well as of their child's strengths, and begin to focus on practical ways of coping.

The above account is based on the reactions most often observed when the parents' discovery of the disability is sudden; as might typically occur, for example, following the birth of a child with a severe mental or physical disability.

The type of feelings parents experience following the diagnosis of Tourette syndrome may be rather different, however. In the first place, since Tourette syndrome may not be diagnosed until the child is at least eight or nine, and often much later (even up to their twenties), there may already have been concerns about his early development for some time before a specialist opinion is sought. As a consequence, many parents already suspect that something may be wrong, so that the news that their child has Tourette syndrome does not come as such a shock, particularly when the siblings appear 'normal'. Nevertheless, even when parents have suspected it, the final confirmation of the diagnosis can still come as a hard blow. 'I'm so shocked,' said a father recently. He and his wife had been seeing specialists for about three years as their son's diagnosis was very complex, but the final and definite confirmation of Tourette syndrome (with ADHD and conduct disorder, in this case) was extremely upsetting for them.

Another reaction, however, is one of relief. 'At least the condition has a name and it proves that my child is not "bad" or "mad,"' said a mother recently. Her child had been going from specialist to specialist and undergoing many investigations. All had proven negative and his conduct was therefore dubbed as 'a behavioural problem'. The relief for this family was that he was not, in fact, 'a bad boy'—he just couldn't help his symptoms.

Many parents feel relief for another reason. Children with Tourette syndrome look normal, and have no particular facial characteristics or features. Therefore most people assume that they are normal and are just badly behaved, often blaming the 'frazzled' parents for rearing the child badly. The parents often say 'At last we can tell people that our son has a recognisable condition' and feel that they are less likely to be blamed.

Another family, however, reacted very differently. When young Peter was diagnosed as having Tourette syndrome, and we explained that it was due to dopamine malfunctioning or 'going wrong' in a certain area of the brain, they were horrified. 'Please don't tell us he's mad', they begged. We had a lot of work explaining how Tourette syndrome was *not* a sign of madness; although dopamine is also involved in schizophrenia (and indeed medications which are given for schizophrenia and Tourette syndrome (although in different doses) both block dopamine), Tourette syndrome and schizophrenia are *not* related.

Other factors may also affect the way in which parents react. For example, the severity of the motor and vocal tics of Tourette syndrome, and the degree of accompanying behavioural disturbances may influence how they respond to the news. In addition, the psychological resilience of each parent, and the amount of support available from their family, friends, and health professionals will also be important, helping some parents to pass through certain stages in their emotional reaction to the diagnosis more quickly than others.

In view of the fact that different people may pass through these stages at different rates or in a different order, it is important to recognize that those members of the family who have not just heard the diagnosis may be at a different stage from those who have known for a while, and that their reactions may continue to be different for some time. They can help each other by showing their feelings. Couples may find it helpful to set aside regular times when they can discuss their worries, frustrations, and sadness together. Brothers and sisters may be jealous of the extra attention and time being devoted to the sibling with Tourette syndrome, not understanding that he or she is basically 'unwell' at some level. For instance, if a classmate at school swears, he or she gets into trouble. The child's sibling might well wonder 'why does my brother or sister not get into trouble for swearing, but just gets attention?'. This situation is difficult to explain to a young brother or sister, but parents should try patiently. Some siblings become sensitive, brave advocates for their brothers and sisters with Tourette syndrome, both at school and in the world outside the family.

Extreme reactions

Sometimes individuals get 'stuck' in certain stages of coping with news such as a diagnosis, or miss some out altogether, and this may lead to difficulties. Thus, parents who cannot accept their child's medical condition may embark on a relentless search for a 'cure', by constantly seeking opinions from many specialists, but never feeling satisfied with the outcome. Continued searching for what might help the child is, of course, both important and valuable. However, extreme reactions are often based more on the parents' need to stave off the sad reality of their own plight, rather than on the child's needs.

Other parents may get caught up in an unresolved phase of anger, becoming embroiled in protracted legal battles with professionals whom they hold somehow responsible for their child's medical condition. Again, valid legal redress is important; but extreme reactions are often based on the need to 'blame' someone. Another legalistic response is to ask the doctor if he or she thinks that the previous doctor who failed to diagnose their child as having Tourette syndrome was guilty of medical negligence. Our opinion is that it is not. For a doctor not to diagnose a fairly rare condition is *not* negligence.

Distinguishing between normal and extreme emotional reactions to the diagnosis is not always straightforward. The distress and feelings of sadness that some parents experience may occasionally precipitate a severe depression in a predisposed individual. By depression we do not mean ordinary feelings of sadness, but rather a depressive illness, a profound misery, with frequent crying, and an inability to derive pleasure from activities that would normally be enjoyable. Often, such depression also involves feelings of pessimism, worthlessness, and excessive guilt, as well as disturbed sleep and appetite, and may be accompanied by feelings of weariness and low energy. Parents may also experience difficulty concentrating or paying attention and feel a sense of numbness—leading to a vicious circle of guilt as they are aware of their child's need for attention and affection, yet they sense that the child knows they are unable to supply it. If this occurs, parents may benefit from professional help, either in the form of counselling, or antidepressant medication, or both. If this is a problem for you or your partner, you should ask your family doctor for help.

As we said earlier, most parents make a remarkable adaptation to their child's needs and problems. Actually, the process of trying to understand their child's problem often brings with it a special intimacy, which comes from the feeling that this is a special child, who needs far more than most children, and with whom one can develop a unique relationship.

Effects on your marriage or relationship

Given the added pressures of raising a child with a condition such as Tourette syndrome, it is small wonder that people often say that having a child with a disability makes or breaks a marriage or relationship. It may be reassuring, then, to learn that parents of children with Tourette syndrome are probably no more likely to separate and divorce than parents of children without disabilities. Nevertheless, difficulties in the relationship may arise, and when this happens it is important to tackle them. Often no more is required of the parents than to set aside time for themselves as partners (rather than just as parents) when they can talk openly, and share and discuss difficulties and disappointments. To find time to do this may not be easy; but the time is well worth the investment. If it is a problem to arrange for friends or relatives to help with the child-care, then the parents should discuss this with one of the professionals.

Another problem in the relationship may occur if one side of the family is blamed for carrying the 'Tourette gene'. This accusation can be very harmful to a relationship. If there were any problems in the parental relationship beforehand, they may be exacerbated as one parent, in despair, blames the other for 'giving' the child the 'bad gene'. This is of course not helpful. None of us can choose which genes we pass on to our children, and inheritance involves a lot of unpredictable factors. Nevertheless, when we are at the end of our tether we can say things that we later regret. It is often said that in despair, you may hurt those who mean the most to you.

Effects on other children in the family

If there are other children in the family, parents will have to tell them of their brother's or sister's Tourette syndrome. Precisely what is said will depend on the age of the particular child and his or her ability to grasp the information. The news may also be a source of distress to them, and will need to be shared in a sensitive manner. It is important to pace what you say, so that your child is able to take the news on board and come to terms with it. It is not enough to have a one-off 'heart to heart' talk and then leave it at that. There will be a host of questions that youngsters will have about the problems of having Tourette syndrome. Parents should discuss these issues openly, to prevent children 'bottling up' their feelings and questions. Ideally, parents should strive to set aside time for siblings so that they know they can ask any questions which are on their minds.

At present not much is known regarding the longer-term effects on development for siblings of children with conditions such as Tourette syndrome, although it does seem that the effects need not be negative, and, indeed, may be positive. Thus, some of the research in this area has indicated that siblings of children with disabilities may develop a deeper understanding of people and of medical conditions in general; they may show more compassion, and have a better appreciation of their own good health than their peers.

On the other hand, some siblings do seem to have problems in emotional adjustment and well-being. This is all the more so, as they may mistakenly fear 'catching' the syndrome from their brother or sister—and of course, they are more at risk of inheriting the Tourette syndrome spectrum than a member of the general population. Siblings also have their own needs and, as far as possible, need time given to them to foster their own development. Parents need to be particularly alert to any hesitation their other children have in inviting friends home. With younger children, it may be sensible for parents to talk with schoolfriends' parents to pave the way for having the friend to visit.

From our experience in the clinic, we understand that both children with Tourette syndrome and their brothers or sisters are particularly vulnerable to bullying and teasing. Tourette syndrome is an easy target for bullying, by the very nature of the condition. We know one patient, a little boy, who is cruelly called the The Syndrome Kid at school, which needless to say saddens him greatly. There is also an added pressure on siblings to protect their brother or sister from bullying or teasing.

Telling a child with Tourette syndrome about his or her condition

Many children with Tourette syndrome may ask why they are different from other children, and parents may have to explain to them that they have a problem, what this means, and how it affects their lives. This is no easy task. Broadly speaking, the same approach we have advocated for siblings is appropriate here. For a start, parents need to be aware of the issues, provide a suitable forum for discussion, share information at a pace appropriate for their child, and pitch the content of what they say at a level that can be understood.

Understandably, children who recognize their disabilities may become troubled by their condition as its impact on their lives becomes more evident. This may occur as a young child, but usually happens during adolescence and early adult life, when problems may arise in establishing and keeping friendships despite wishes to the contrary. Marked

unhappiness (and even depressive illness) occasionally may develop as a consequence. If this does
emerge, parents should seek professional advice for
their son or daughter. A few children with severe
Tourette syndrome have said that they would rather
be dead than cope with the 'twitches' forever.

Other individuals, however, cope by treating their
disorder with fondness. Some individuals call it 'my
syndrome', and find this comforting. An adult patient
of ours calls it her 'G & T'. A young girl patient of
ours calls her coprolia Ethel.

Talking about the problems to friends and relatives

In addition to telling siblings, parents will also have
to let their own parents and families know that their
child has Tourette syndrome. It is as well to bear in
mind that the news may be distressing for grand-
parents although they may feel uneasy about sharing
their distress. One particular area that some families
feel sensitive about, and which can cause difficulty,
concerns the possible hereditary factors involved in
the syndrome. It is important in this respect for
families to be aware of the relevant information
while not getting caught up in unhelpful recrimina-
tions like 'it's not on our side of the family'.

The issues are complex, and other close relatives
planning a family may find it helpful to seek the
advice of an expert in genetic counselling. We know
of one case where after hearing that Tourette syndrome is genetic, a mother requested a termination of
her next pregnancy, which was granted. Unfortunately in this case, no clear genetic counselling
was sought, which might have made the couple

consider their choices in the light of all the information available. Had she discussed it with appropriate professionals in more detail, she might not have chosen to have the termination.

Much the same advice about talking to relatives also holds when dealing with friends and acquaintances—it is important to openly provide straightforward information about the child's disorder. This is the most effective way of preventing misunderstandings caused by ignorance or prejudice. This is, however, often easier said than done. It can sometimes be quite challenging to think of ways of answering the critical looks or comments that parents may get when their child behaves strangely in public, such as swearing inappropriately and out of the blue, or being hyperactive and constantly running about and climbing on to things. For advice on how to tackle these sorts of problems, other parents of children with Tourette syndrome may often have useful ideas. For a novel introductory card, see Appendix 1.

Indeed, because of this, we often recommend that parents and patients join the Tourette Syndrome Association and thus find support from parents and individuals who have similar problems. Judgement needs to exercised of course; if the child, for example, is an uncomplicated case, parents do not always do well by contacting parents whose children have much more complex problems. We usually discuss the pros and cons of joining the association, tailoring the discussion to the individuals concerned. In the UK the Tourette Syndrome Association has a telephone help-line that serves families during the working week. The UK and USA associations also have 'Question and Answer' leaflets. These are professional and authoritative, and some people with Tourette syndrome carry these leaflets with them ready to offer to those who ask awkward questions! In the Tourette Syndrome Associations there are also local area groups (chapters) who have meetings and support groups. Joining an organisation such as the Tourette Syndrome Association can lead to discovering lots of practical tips, such as names of hotels that have an understanding and progressive policy towards people with disabilities—making holidays that much easier. They can give advice on benefits and other entitlements as well. By making contact with other individuals in the same situation, one can learn how they are coping and, in that way, feel less isolated or overwhelmed by one's own situation. Some parents even begin to believe that, with others, they can work to make the world a better place not only for their own child, but for all children and individuals with Tourette syndrome.

5
Education and Tourette syndrome: what can be done?

How common are tics and Tourette syndrome in schoolchildren?

Tics occur in around 10 to 20 percent of school age children; however, as we said in chapter 2, the accepted prevalence of Tourette syndrome is much lower, at around one in 2000. It is also unclear what proportion of children who have tics actually have Tourette syndrome or one of the other tic disorders. It should be noted that prevalence figures are likely to be underestimates, as they are based on clinic or other special populations (which usually focus on a disproportionate number of severe or complex cases). That is, the mild cases may be overlooked because they do not come to medical attention.

In addition to tics, Tourette syndrome can be associated, as we have said in earlier chapters, with symptoms such as coprophenomena (uttering obscene words or making obscene gestures), echophenomena (copying behaviours), or behaviour disturbances such as self-injury, or obsessive–compulsive behaviour, and attention deficit hyperactivity disorder. Taken together, this spectrum of clinical problems commonly contributes to school problems in children with Tourette syndrome.

The only published studies to date have come from the USA and UK. The first study found that up to a third of children with Tourette syndrome experienced learning problems including learning disability (22 percent), needing to repeat a grade (12 percent), poor grades (18 percent) and full time special education classes (12 percent). Another group studied students referred for educational assessment in a Californian district, and reported that as many as 12 percent of all children referred had Tourette syndrome and 28 percent had a broader tic disorder diagnosis.

In a community-based study using direct clinical examination, another group found that, of the special education population, 26 percent had definite or probable tics as compared to 6 percent of regular classroom students. We have conducted two investigations in schools in the United Kingdom examining children for tics and Tourette syndrome and have found many more cases than expected, especially in children with educational problems. All these figures together suggest that not only is Tourette syndrome in children more common than was once thought, but also that it may well be over-represented in special education populations.

What problems do children with Tourette syndrome have at school?

Children with Tourette syndrome may have difficulties in education for a variety of reasons, including the tics themselves, specific learning difficulties, the associated behaviours of obsessive–compulsive behaviour (OCB), or attention deficit hyperactivity disorder (ADHD), or the side effects of medication.

It must be restated that, in our opinion, the majority of mild cases of Tourette syndrome are probably unknown to health professionals, and are well-adjusted people living in the community. To date, no studies have been conducted on the psychological and educational profiles of such people. They may have subtle difficulties in learning that do not affect their overall performance and therefore need no extra help with their education. We have diagnosed Tourette syndrome in adults who have become doctors, lawyers, accountants, teachers, armed forces personnel. In fact, for people working in all sorts of professions, aspects of Tourette syndrome (eg obsessionality) may actually be a strength, not a disability. For example, an obsessional accountant may be known as meticulous and careful. Any of us would surely want to consult such a person.

Some children with Tourette syndrome may encounter problems at school. First, some tics, such as severe head-shaking, neck-stretching or eye-rolling, may render the child unable to look straight at the teacher for a continuous length of time, or render them unable to read easily, and this can obviously cause educational problems. Similarly, hand tics may interfere with writing, making it untidy or even illegible. Loud and complex vocalizations may interrupt the flow of speech, or disturb the other children in class. Thus the education not only of the child with Tourette syndrome, but possibly that of their peers may also be affected. This in turn may have difficult ramifications for the child him or herself.

Whilst studies of children with Tourette syndrome have usually reported the distribution of intelligence (IQ) to be normal, some 'visuospatial deficits' have been documented. These may cause problems such as difficulty with copying things, which children are required to do in a variety of settings, (eg doing homework, or when copying from books or the blackboard). Children with Tourette syndrome may also have problems with attention and impulsiveness, even if they do not have the full ADHD diagnosis.

Those children however who have the associated behaviours of OCB and ADHD will be much more disadvantaged. Children with obsessions may become pedantic in their talk, have a need for strict routine, a need for absolute perfection and having everything 'just right'. This may interfere with a homework assignment, as they may be compelled to do it over and over again, until it is 'just right', at the expense of other assignments which they are unable to do for lack of sufficient time. We have seen several children who literally take hours to do their homework—way in excess of normal, and often they may never complete it. They may also be slow in their work, through always trying to be perfect. Such children may engage in rituals, which prevent them getting on with their school work or home work.

Children with both Tourette syndrome and additional ADHD have very special problems. As we stated earlier, ADHD is characterized by poor attention, poor concentration, being easily distracted, fidgeting, hyperactivity, and impulsiveness. Hence, these children often fail to give close attention to detail, or make careless mistakes in their schoolwork or homework. They often have difficulty in maintaining their attention, on school work, or even on enjoyable things such as playing.

Often, they appear not to be listening when spoken to, and thus they may not actually absorb information, which obviously causes problems. They may also have difficulty in finishing tasks such as schoolwork or homework. They may have special difficulties in organising things, and may lose things such as toys or their school things (pens, pencils, rubbers (erasers), rulers, books etc). They may appear easily distracted, and their work or stream of thought may be interrupted by hearing someone outside the classroom, such as in the playground, to whom they may pay more attention than to what is going on in the lesson. They may also cause them to be forgetful and thus not do their homework or other tasks which have been set for them.

The hyperactivity is also characterized by fidgeting, leaving their desk in the classroom repeatedly, running about or climbing on things. A hyperactive child in the clinic can cause mayhem—and for the teachers at school things can be worse. They have a class of 30 or so to deal with, so a child who is hyperactive may cause chaos and needs specific assistance. Children with ADHD may also be noisy, talk too much or appear always 'on the go'. Their impulsiveness can be demonstrated by their butting into other people's conversations, or answering questions directed at other children in the class.

We see an increasing number of children with Tourette syndrome in the clinic who also have *conduct disorder*. Children with conduct disorder show inappropriate and sometimes severe aggression to people and animals and may, for example, starting physical fights in the playground. They may be very destructive. Some children set fires deliberately, they may lie often, or steal, and might run away from home or play truant from school. Needless to say, these children are especially difficult to deal with at school. Setting boundaries (that is, saying very clearly what is and what is not acceptable) is important, and these must be reinforced with firm but kind discipline. There is an association between ADHD and conduct disorder and, as mentioned earlier, unfortunately some of these children grow up to develop what is known as a *personality disorder*. If a child does have these characteristics, it is imperative for the parents to obtain expert advice about management, since otherwise the long term outlook may not be good. While in the clinic we see many adult Tourette syndrome patients with personality disorders, in our experience few end up with serious criminal records. Once again, the incidence of these problems in individuals with mild Tourette syndrome in the community is unknown, but we would not expect it to be high.

Finally, there are the possible side-effects of medication which may, regrettably, affect learning. For example, medications such as sulpiride, haloperidol, and pimozide may all cause sedation at some level, which might in turn affect the child's concentration. These medications can also cause blurring of vision, which may make reading difficult, although this is not common with the low doses given in Tourette syndrome. There have even been a few reports that some of these medications have caused school phobia and school refusal, but these are, thankfully, rare. Some medications may also cause depression which could make a child irritable, down, and not willing to learn. Methylphenidate is sometimes given to children with Tourette syndrome who also have ADHD in the UK, but it is much more frequently prescribed in the USA and Australia. While it can reduce the hyperactivity and improve poor concentration, it may increase the actual motor and vocal tics, and some children who take it also lose weight.

Children with Tourette syndrome obviously need to be understood. While they may be able to suppress their tics voluntarily, often at the expense of a build up of inner tension, they do not 'put them on'. The tics are not strictly under voluntary control. Suppression may result in an increase in rebound tics and may cause children social embarrassment. For this reason, attention should not be drawn to the tics. Teachers should be informed of the tics and behaviours, however, so that they may see the child in terms of his having a recognized disability, rather than being naughty. Unfortunately, as we have said, we have seen cases of children being teased and bullied because of their tics and noises. We believe that some children with Tourette syndrome require special educational assistance (see below).

What can be achieved?

Hopefully, most children with Tourette syndrome will eventually attain the grades and education that are expected of them. Of course, some do fall behind their peers, especially when they have ADHD, but most actually achieve acceptable goals. An apt reminder of what can be achieved by individuals with Tourette syndrome is the surgeon Dr Mort Doran (who is also an aeroplane pilot), and the other doctors described in Dr Oliver Sacks book *An Anthropologist on Mars* (see Chapter 4). We also have many patients with higher education and degrees.

Statement of special educational needs

In the UK and many other countries, children with problems require a Statement of their educational needs. This Statement is prepared by an educational psychologist, in order to recognize and formalize the provision of special educational help, such as a place in a special school, or a personal assistant teacher in a mainstream school. Following an evaluation, the educational psychologist and other professionals involved in the child's care compile a report for the local education authority. This sets the wheels in motion for access to the most suitable school or education for that particular child. When the Statementing runs smoothly, it is a good way of ensuring the best for a child and keeping the child's needs under review. Parents are invited to comment on and contribute to the draft Statement before it is finalized, so that they should not feel inhibited about expressing their concerns and views.

It should be noted that parents may experience difficulty at this stage, sometimes because the professionals have a different view of their child's educational needs, or more commonly, because the process may be so protracted, with families perhaps having to fight bureaucracy at every stage. Another frequent disappointment is what has become known as 'resource-led Statementing', meaning that the Statement may be written only with a view to what funding is locally available, rather than to what the child actually needs. Parents should therefore read the Statement carefully to check that they agree with the details of the evaluation. We hope that the system will become easier for parents to use.

It is a source of exasperation that they can well do without.

If the local education authority decides not to Statement a child for special educational needs, they write a 'note in lieu of Statement' which sets out the reasons for their decision not to make a Statement after the assessment.

Can doctor's letters help?

We often write to schools and teachers suggesting that the child receives a Statement or, if not, we recommend measures which could help the child get better access the curriculum. These measures may include one-to-one tuition at times, extra time for examinations or for completing assignments, using a calculator for mathematics, taking examinations in a separate room, and writing the examinations on a computer. If the child has additional ADHD and is disruptive, he may require 'time out' out of class to give his peers and the teachers a break. We point out however, that this 'time out' must in no way be punitive, as the symptoms are beyond the child's control. We also explain to the educators that we often prescribe medication for the children, which hopefully will reduce the disturbing symptoms.

What else can help?

The Tourette Syndrome Associations in the UK and the USA have video films about people with Tourette syndrome. Some schools and teachers find them useful for themselves as well as for the peers of the child with the syndrome. In this way other students can develop tolerance and understanding. In addition, the Tourette Syndrome Associations have literature targeted at schools, and teachers are welcome to attend Association meetings.

Many children with Tourette syndrome enjoy sport and problems with tics and behaviour are often improved (ie, less severe or frequent) during these activities. Ironically, the children are often better when they are concentrating hard on a task. Thus, we encourage participation in sport, if the child enjoys it, as this may be an area in which they may succeed and improve their self-esteem. A mentioned earlier, in America there is a famous baseball player, Jim Eisenreich, who has Tourette syndrome, and he has been a great inspiration to both children and adults with Tourette syndrome.

This reinforces our key message: encourage the child with Tourette syndrome to concentrate on his or her strengths, and give them an extra large dose of praise and encouragement for those activities. Children (and adults) with Tourette syndrome may lack self-esteem and confidence. Therefore, when they manage to suppress tics at an important time (eg during a concert) or when they do well at a particular task, this should be congratulated or acknowledged. This can increase their sense of self-worth, encourage them and help them, and us to focus not just on their condition, but on them, their achievements, and individual contributions.

Appendix 1
An introductory card

One Tourette sufferer has a novel way of introducing himself in new situations such as on an aeroplane, bus, or in a restaurant.

 Hi! My name is Paul

You may receive this card as a friend, employer or fellow student. As I have a visible and at times vivid neurological disorder, TOURETTE SYNDROME, I find this an easy, quick and necessary medium of introduction.

T.S. basically consists of involuntary movements and vocalisations - including obscenities. Symptoms can appear as outbursts.

All I ask is for you to see beyond Tourette to someone who in all other ways is normal and in many ways loves and excels at life.

PAUL M. SMITH - President, W.A. Tourette Syndrome Org (Inc.)

Appendix 2
Bibliography

We have provided a list of references to the scientific literature for interested readers, under *keyword* headings. We hope this will be useful for health professionals and students, whilst not being off-putting to sufferers and their families. We must point out that this is not an exhaustive list of references, but a guide with many key references under each heading.

Worldwide accepted diagnostic criteria

American Psychiatric Association (1994). *Diagnostic and Statistical Manual of Mental Disorders* (4th edition) (DSM IV). American Psychiatric Association, Washington DC.

World Health Organization (1992). *International classification of diseases and health related problems*—(Tenth Revision). World Health Organization, Geneva.

Historical aspects and famous people who may have had Tourette syndrome

Gilles De La Tourette, G. (1885). Etude sur une affection nerveuse caracterisée par de l'incoordination motrice accompagnée d'echolalie et de copralalie. *Archives of Neurology*, **9**, 19–42, 158–200.

Hurst, M.J. and Hurst, D.L. (1994). Tolstoy's description of Tourette syndrome in Anna Karenina. *Journal of Child Neurology*, **94**, 366–67.

Itard, J.M.G. (1825). Memoire sur quelques fonctions involontaires des appareils de la locomotion de la préhension et de la voix. *Archives General Medicine*, **8**, 385–407.

Lees, A.J. (1986). Georges Gilles de la Tourette: the man and his times. *Revue Neurologique* (Paris), **142**, 11, 808–16.

McHenry, L.C. Jr (1967). Samuel Johnson's tics and gesticulations. *Journal of the History of Medicine*, **22**, 152–68.

Meige, H. and Feindel, E. (1907) Tics and Their Treatment. *in* Wilson, S.A.K (ed and transl). William Wood and Company, New York.

Murray, T.J. (1979). Dr. Samuel Johnson's movement disorder. *British Medical Journal*, **1**, 1610–14.

Robertson, M.M. and Reinstein, D.Z. (1991). Convulsive tic disorder. Georges Gilles de la Tourette, Guinon and Grasset on the phenomenology and psychopathology of the Gilles de la Tourette syndrome. *Behavioural Neurology*, **4**, 29–56.

Simkin, B. (1992). Mozart's scatological disorder. *British Medical Journal*, **305**, (6868), 1563–66.

Epidemiology: how common are tics and Tourette syndrome?

Apter, A. *et al.* (1993). An epidemiologic study of Gilles de la Tourette's syndrome in Israel. *Archives of General Psychiatry*, **9**, 734–8.

Burd, L., Kerbeshian, J., Fisher, W. (1986). Prevalence of Gilles de la Tourette syndrome in North Dakota adults. *American Journal of Psychiatry*, **143**, 787–8.

Caine, E.D., *et al.* (1988). Tourette syndrome in Monroe county school children. *Neurology*, **38**, 472–5.

Comings, D.E., Himes, J.A., Comings, B.G. (1990). An epidemiological study of Tourette syndrome in a single school district. *Journal of Clinical Psychiatry*, **51**, 463–9.

Eapen, V., Robertson, M.M., Zeitlin, H., Kurlan, R. (1997) Gilles de la Tourette's Syndrome. *In* Special Education Schools: A United Kingdom Study. *Journal of Neurology*, **244**, 378–82.

Fallon, T. and Schwab–Stone, M. (1992). Methodology of Epidemiological Studies of Tic Disorders and Comorbid Psychopathology. *In* Chase, T.N., Friedhoff, A.J., Cohen, D.J. (eds): *Tourette Syndrome: Genetics, Neurobiology and Treatment. Advances in Neurology*, Vol. 58, pp. 43–55. Raven Press, New York.

Kerbeshian, J. and Burd, L. (1992). The North Dakota prevalence studies of Tourette syndrome and other developmental disorders. In T.N. Chase, A.J. Friedhoff, D.J. Cohen (eds), *Tourette syndrome: genetics, neurobiology and treatment, advances in neurology*, Vol. 58, pp.67–74. New York, Raven Press.

Kurlan, R. (1992). Tourette syndrome in a special education population. In T.N. Chase, A.J. Friedhoff, D.J. Cohen (eds): *Tourette syndrome: genetics, neurobiology and treatment, advances in neurology*, Vol. 58, pp. 75–81. New York, Raven Press.

Kurlan, R. et al. (1994). Tourette's syndrome in a special education population: a pilot study involving a single school district. *Neurology*, **44**, 699–702.

Shapiro, E. (1981). Tic disorders. *Journal of the American Medical Association*, **245**, 1583–5.

Zohar, A.H., et al.. (1992). An epidemiological study of obsessive–compulsive disorder and related disorders in Israeli adolescents. *Journal of the American Academy of Child and Adolescent Psychiatry*, **31**, 1057–61.

Clinical characteristics

Bliss, J. (1980). Sensory experiences of Gilles de la Tourette syndrome. *Archives of General Psychiatry*, **37**, 1343–7.

Cohen, D.J. and Leckman, J.F. (1992). Sensory phenomena associated with Gilles de la Tourette syndrome. *Journal of Clinical Psychiatry*, 53, 319–93.

Eapen, V., Moriarty, J., and Robertson, M.M. (1994). Stimulus induced behaviours in Tourette syndrome? *Journal of Neurology, Neurosurgery and Psychiatry*, **57**, 853–55.

Jankovic, J. and Stone, L. (1991). Dystonic tics in patients with Tourette's syndrome. *Movement Disorders*, **6**(3), 248–52.

Kurlan, R. et al. (1996). Non-obscene complex socially inapproopriate behaviour in Tourette syndrome. *Journal of Neuropsychiatry and Clinical Neursciences*, **8**, 311–17.

Leckman, J.F., Walker, D.E., and Cohen, D.J. (1993). Premonitory urges in Tourette's syndrome. *American Journal of Psychiatry*, **150**, 98–102.

Leckman, J.F., Walker, D.E., Goodman, W.K. et al. (1994). 'Just right' perceptions associated with compulsive behavior in Tourette's syndrome. *American Journal of Psychiatry*, **151**, 675–80.

Moriarty, J., Ring, H.A., and Robertson, M.M. (1993). An *idiot savant* calendrical calculator with Gilles de la Tourette syndrome: implications for an understanding of the *savant* syndrome. *Psychological Medicine*, **23**, 1019–21.

Robertson, M.M., Trimble, M.R. and Lees, A.J. (1989). Self-injurious behaviour and the Gilles de la Tourette syndrome: a clinical study and review of the literature. *Psychological Medicine*, **19**, 611–25.

Sachdev, P., Chee, K.Y. and Wilson, A. (1996). Tics status. *Australian and New Zealand Journal of Psychiatry*, **30**, 392–96.

The long term outcome

Bruun, R.D. *et al* (1976). A follow-up of 78 patients with Gilles de la Tourette syndrome. *American Journal of Psychiatry*, **133**, 944–7.

Carter, A.S. *et al.* (1994). A prospective longitudinal study of Gilles de la Tourette syndrome. *Journal of the American Academy of Child and Adolescent Psychiatry*, **33**, 377–85.

Erenberg, G. *et al.* (1987). The natural history of Tourette syndrome: a follow-up study. *Annals of Neurology*, **22**, 383–5.

Musisi, S. *et al.* (1990). Gilles de la Tourette syndrome. A follow-up study. *Journal of Clinical Pharmacology*, **3**, 197–9.

Psychopathology and psychiatric aspects

Golden, G.S. (1984). Psychologic and neuropsychologic aspects of Tourette's syndrome. *Neurologic Clinics*, **21**, 91–102.

Robertson, M.M., Trimble, M.R., and Lees, A.J. (1988). The psychopathology of the Gilles de la Tourette syndrome: a phenomenological analysis. *British Journal of Psychiatry*, **152**, 383–90.

Robertson, M.M. *et al.* (1993). The psychopathology of Gilles de la Tourette syndrome: a controlled study. *British Journal of Psychiatry*, **162**, 114–17.

Robertson, M.M., Eapen, V., and Van de Wetering, B.J.M. (1995). Suicide in Gilles de la Tourette syndrome—a report of two cases. *Journal of Clinical Psychiatry*, **56**, 8, 378.

Robertson, M.M. *et al.* (1977). Personality disorder and psychopathology in Tourette's syndrome: A controlled study. *British Journal of Psychiatry*, **171**, 283–6.

Stefl, M.E. (1984). Mental health needs associated with Tourette's syndrome. *American Journal of Public Health*, **74**, 1313.

Neuropsychology and psychological testing and education

Baron-Cohen, A.S. and Robertson, M.M. (1995). Children with either autism, Gilles de la Tourette syndrome, or both: mapping cognition to specific syndromes. *Neurocase*, **1**, 101–4.

Baron-Cohen, S. *et al.* (1994). Can children with Gilles de la Tourette syndrome edit their intentions? *Psychological Medicine*, **24**, 29–40.

Bornstein, R.A. (1990). Neuropsychological performance in children with Tourette's syndrome. *Psychiatry Research*, **33**, 73–81.

Brookshire, B.L. *et al.* (1994). Neuropsychological characteristics of children with Tourette syndrome: evidence for a nonverbal learning disability. *Journal of Clinical and Experimental Neuropsychology*, **16**, 289–302.

Channon, S., Flynn, D., and Robertson, M.M. (1992). Attentional deficits in Gilles de la Tourette syndrome. *Neuropsychiatry, Neuropsychology, and Behavioral Neurology*, **5**, 170–7.

Dykens, E.M. *et al.* (1990). Intellectual, academic, and adaptive functioning of Tourette's syndrome children with and without attention deficit disorder. *Journal of Abnormal Child Psychiatry*, **18**, 607–14.

Georgiou, N. *et al.* (1995). The Simon effect and attention deficits in Gilles de La Tourette's syndrome and Huntington's disease. *Brain*, **118** (5), 1305–18.

Georgiou, N. *et al.* (1996). The effect of Huntington's disease and Gilles de la Tourette syndrome on the ability to hold and shift attention. *Neuropsychologia*, **34**, 843–51.

Oades, R.D. *et al.* (1996). Auditory event-related potentials (ERPs) and mismatch negativity (MMN) in healthy children and those with attention-deficit or Tourette/tic symptoms. *Biological Psychology*, **43**, 163–85.

Schuerholz, L.J. *et al.* (1996). Neuropsychological status of children with Tourette's Sydnrome with and without attention deficit hyperactivity disorder. *Neurology*, **46**, 958–65.

Tourette syndrome and obsessive-compulsive disorder

Cath, D.C. *et al.* (1992). Mental play in Gilles de la Tourette's syndrome and obsessive–compulsive disorder. *British Journal of Psychiatry*, **161**, 542–5.

de Groot, C.M. *et al.* (1995). Patterns of obsessive compulsive symptoms in Tourette subjects are independent of severity. *Anxiety*, **1**, 268–74.

Frankel, M. *et al.* (1986). Obsessions and compulsions in Gilles de la Tourette's syndrome. *Neurology*, **36**, 378–82.

George, M.S. *et al.* (1993). Obsessions in obsessive–compulsive disorder (OCD) with and without Gilles de la Tourette syndrome. *American Journal of Psychiatry*, **150**, 93–7.

Holzer, J.C., Goodman, W.K., and McDougle, C.J. (1994). Obsessive-compulsive disorder with and without a chronic tic disorder. *British Journal of Psychiatry*, **164**, 469–73.

Leonard, H.L. *et al.* (1992). Tourette syndrome and obsessive–compulsive disorder. *In* T.N. Chase, A.J. Friedhoff, and D.J. Cohen (eds), *Tourette syndrome: genetics, neurobiology and treatment, advances in neurology*, Vol 58, pp 83–93. New York, Raven Press.

Miguel, E.C. *et al.* (1995). Phenomenology of intentional repetitive behaviours in obsessive–compulsive disorder and Tourette's syndrome. *Journal of Clinical Psychiatry*, **56**, 246–55.

Robertson, M.M. (1995). The relationship between Gilles de la Tourette syndrome and obsessive compulsive disorder. *Journal of Serotonin Research*, **Suppl 1**, 49–62.

Robertson, M.M. and Yakeley, J. (1993). Obsessive-compulsive and self injurious behaviour. *In* R. Kurlan (ed.), *Handbook of Tourette's syndrome and related tic and behavioural disorders*, pp 45–87. Marcel Dekker. New York .

Santangelo, S.L., Pauls, D.L., and Goldstein, J.M. (1994). Tourette's syndrome: What are the influences of gender and comorbid obsessive–compulsive disorder? *Journal of the American Academy of Child and Adolescent Psychiatry*, **33**, 795–804.

Aetiology: Suggested causes of Tourette's syndrome

Neuroanatomy and neurophysiology

Balthasar, K. (1957). Uber das anatomische Substrat der generalisierten Tic-Krankheit (maladie des tics, Gilles de la Tourette): Entwicklungshemmung des Corpus striatum. *Archiv für Psychiatrie und Nervenkrankheiten*, **195**, 531–49.

Cohen, D.J., and Leckman, J.F. (1994). Developmental psychopathology and neurobiology of Tourette's syndrome. *Journal of the American Academy of Child and Adolescent Psychiatry*, **33**, 2–15.

Devinsky, O. (1983). Neuroanatomy of Gilles de la Tourette's syndrome: possible midbrain involvement. *Archives of Neurology*, **40**, 508–14.

Dewulf, A., van Bogaert, L. (1941) Etudes anatomo-cliniques de syndromes hypercinetique complexes—Partie 3. Une observation anatomo-clinique de maladie des tics (Gilles de la Tourette). *Monatsschrift für Psychiatrie und Neurologie*, **104**, 53–61.

Haber, S.N. *et al.* (1986). Gilles de la Tourette's syndrome. A postmortem neuropathological and immunohistochemical study. *Journal of the Neurological Sciences*, **75**, 225–41.

Haber, S.N. and Wolfer, D. (1992). Basal ganglia peptidergic staining in Tourette syndrome. *In* Chase, T.N., Friedhoff, A.J., Cohen, D.J. (eds) *Tourette syndrome: genetics, neurobiology and treatment, advances in neurology*, Vol. 58, pp. 145–50. Raven Press, New York.

Obeso, J.A., Rothwell, J.C, and Marsden, C.D. (1982). The neurophysiology of Tourette syndrome. *In*: A.J. Friedhoff and T.N. Chase (eds) Gilles de la Tourette syndrome, *Advances in Neurology*, pp.105–114. Raven Press, New York.

Rickards, H., Dursun, S.M., and Farrar, G. (1996). Increased plasma kynurenine and its relationship to neopterin and tryptophan in Tourette's syndrome. *Psychological Medicine*, **26**, 857–62.

Singer, H.S. *et al.* (1982). Dopaminergic dysfunction in Tourette syndrome. *Annals of Neurology*, **12**, 361–6.

Van de Wetering, B.J.M. *et al.* (1985). Late components of the auditory evoked potentials in Gilles de la Tourette syndrome. *Clinics in Neurology and Neurosurgery*, **87**, 181–6.

Genetics and family studies

Kurlan, R. *et al*. (1986). Familial Tourette's syndrome: report of a large pedigree and potential for linkage analysis. *Neurology*, **36**, 772–6.

McMahon, W.M. *et al*. (1992). Tourette symptoms in 161 related family members. *In*: T.N. Chase, A.J. Friedhoff, and D.J. Cohen (eds), *Tourette syndrome: genetics, neurobiology and treatment, advances in neurology*, Vol. 58, pp. 159–65. Raven Press, New York.

Price, R.A., Kidd, K.K., Cohen, D.J. *et al*. (1985). A twin study of Tourette syndrome. *Archives of General Psychiatry*, **42**, 815–20.

Randolph, C. *et al*. (1993). Tourette's syndrome in monozygotic twins. Relationship of tic severity to neuropsychological function. *Archives of Neurology*, **50**, 725–8.

Robertson, M.M. and Gourdie, A. (1990). Familial Tourette's syndrome in a large British pedigree: associated psychopathology, severity, and potential for linkage analysis. *British Journal of Psychiatry*, **156**, 515–21.

Eapen, V., Pauls, D.L., Robertson, M.M. (1993). Evidence for autosomal dominant transmission in Gilles de la Tourette syndrome—United Kingdom cohort. *British Journal of Psychiatry*, **162**, 593–6.

Eapen, V. *et al*. (1997). Sex of parent transmission effect in Tourette's syndrome: evidence for earlier age at onset in maternally transmitted cases suggests a geronomic imprinting effect. *Neurology*, **48**, 934–7.

Kurlan, R. *et al*. (1994). Bilineal transmission in Tourette's syndrome families. *Neurology*, **44**, 2336–42.

Pakstis, A.J. *et al*. (1991). Progress in the search for genetic linkage with Tourette syndrome: an exclusion map covering more than 50 percent of the autosomal genome. *American Journal of Human Genetics*, **48**, 281–94.

Pauls, D.L., Pakstis, A.J., and Kurlan, R. (1990). Segregation and linkage analyses of Gilles de la Tourette's syndrome and related disorders. *Journal of the American Academy of Child and Adolescent Psychiatry*, **29**, 195–203.

Robertson, M.M., and Trimble, M.R. (1993). Normal chromosomal findings in Gilles de la Tourette syndrome. *Psychiatric Genetics* **3**, 95–9.

Other factors in aetiology

Allen, J.A., Leonard, H.L., and Swedo, S.E. (1995). Infection-triggered, autoimmune, subtype of paedatric OCD and Tourette's syndrome. *Journal of the Americal Academy of Child and Adolescent Psychiatry*, **34**, 307–11.

Leckman, J.F. *et al.* (1987). Nongenetic factors in Gilles de la Tourette's syndrome. *Archives of General Psychiatry*, **44**, 100.

Leckman, J.F., Dolnansky, E.S., and Hardin, M.T. (1990). Perinatal factors in the expression of Tourette's syndrome: an exploratory study. *Journal of the American Academy of Child and Adolescent Psychiatry*, **29**, 220–6.

Pulst, S.-M., Walshe, T.M., Romero, J.A. (1983). Carbon monoxide poisoning with features of Gilles de la Tourette's syndrome. *Archives of Neurology*, **40**, 443–4.

Rickards, H., *et al.* (1996). Increased plasma kynurenine and its relationship to neopterin and tryptophan in Tourette's syndrome. *Psychological Medicine*, **26**, 857–62.

Robertson, M.M. *et al.* (1987). Copper abnormalities in the Gilles de la Tourette syndrome. *Biological Psychiatry*, **22**, 968–78.

Iatrogenic—Tourette syndrome following other medications

Klawans, H.L. *et al.* (1978). Gilles de la Tourette syndrome after long-term chlorpromazine therapy. *Neurology (NY)*, **28**, 1064–8.

Mueller, J. and Aminoff, M.J. (1982). Tourette-like syndrome after long-term neuroleptic drug treatment. *British Journal of Psychiatry*, **141**, 191–3.

Allergy

Finegold, I. (1985). Allergy and Tourette's syndrome. *Annals of Allergy*, **55**, 119–21.

Neuroimaging

Braun, A.R. *et al.* (1993). The functional neuroanatomy of Tourette's syndrome: an FDG–PET study. I. Regional changes in cerebral glucose metabolism differentiating patients and controls. *Neuropsychopharmacology*, **9**, 277–91.

George, M.S. *et al.* (1993). Elevated frontal cerebral blood flow in Gilles de la Tourette syndrome: a Tc99HM–PAO SPECT study. Psychiatry Research. *Neuroimaging*, **45**, 143–51.

George, M.S. *et al.* (1994. Dopamine receptor availability in Tourette's syndrome. *Psychiatry Research: Neuroimaging*, **55**, 193–203.

Hyde, T.M., Stacey, M.E., and Coppola, R. (1995). Cerebral morphometric abnormalities in Tourette's syndrome: a quantitative MRI study of monozygotic twins. *Neurology*, **45**, 1176–82.

Malison, R.T., McDougle, C.J., and van Dyck, C.H. (1995). 123I beta-CIT SPECT imaging of striatal dopamine transporter binding in Tourette's disorder. *American Journal of Psychiatry*, **152**, 1359–61.

Moriarty, J. *et al.* (1995). Brain perfusion abnormalities in Gilles de la Tourette's syndrome. *British Journal of Psychiatry* **167**, 249–54.

Peterson, B. *et al.* (1993). Reduced basal ganglia volumes in Tourette's syndrome using three-dimensional reconstruction techniques from magnetic resonance images. *Neurology*, **43**, 941–9.

Singer, H.S. *et al.* (1993). Volumetric MRI changes in basal ganglia of children with Tourette's syndrome. *Neurology*, **43**, 950–6.

Turjanski, N. *et al.* (1994). PET studies of the presynaptic and postsynaptic dopaminergic system in Tourette's syndrome. *Journal of Neurology, Neurosurgery and Psychiatry*, **57**, 688–92.

Wolf, S.S. *et al.* (1996). Tourette syndrome: prediction of phenotypic variation in monozygotic twins by caudate nucleus D2 receptor binding. *Science*, **273**, 1225–7.

Treatment

Medication

Bruun, R.D. (1988). Subtle and underrecognised side effects of neuroleptic treatment in children with Tourette's disorder. *American Journal of Psychiatry*, **145**, 621–4.

Eggers, C.H., Rothenberger, A., and Berghaus, U. (1988). Clinical and neurobiological findings in children suffering from tic disease following treatment with tiapride. *European Archives of Psychiatric and Neurological Sciences*, **237**, 223–9.

Jankovic, J. and Beach, J. (1997). Long-term effects of Tetrabenazine in hyperkinetic movement disorders. *Neurology*, **48**, 358–62.

Leckman, J.F. *et al.* (1985). Short and long-term treatment of Tourette's syndrome with clonidine: a clinical perspective. *Neurology*, **35**, 343–51.

McConville, B.J. *et al.* (1992). The effects of nicotine plus haloperidol compared to nicotine only and placebo nicotine only in reducing tic severity and frequency in Tourette's disorder. *Biological Psychiatry*, **31**, 832–40.

Riddle, M.A. *et al.* (1990) .Fluoxetine treatment of children and adolescents with Tourette's and obsessive compulsive disorders: preliminary clinical experience, *Journal of the American Academy of Child and Adolescent Psychiatry*, **29**, 45–8.

Robertson, M.M., Schnieden, V., and Lees, A.J. (1990). Management of Gilles de la Tourette syndrome using sulpiride. *Clinical Neuropharmacology*, **13**, 229–35.

Robertson, M.M. *et al.* (1996). Risperidone in the treatment of Tourette syndrome—a retrospective case note study. *Journal of Psychopharmacology*, **10**, 317–20.

Sallee, F.R. *et al.* (1997). Relative efficacy of Haloperidol and Pimozide in children and adolescents with Tourette's disorder. *American Journal of Psychiatry*, **154**, 1057–62.

Scott, B.L., Jankovic, J., and Donovan, D.T. (1996). Botulinum toxin injection into vocal cord in the treatment of malignant coprolalia associated with Tourette's syndrome. *Movement Disorders*, **11**, 431–3.

Behavioural treatment

Azrin, N.H. and Peterson, A.L. (1988). Behaviour therapy for Tourette's syndrome. In: D.J. Cohen, R.D. Brown, J.F. Leckman (eds), Tourette syndrome and tic disorders: clinical understanding and treatment, pp.237–55. John Wiley, New York

Neurosurgical treatment

Baer, L., Rauch, S.L., and Jenike, M.A. (1994). Cingulotomy in a case of concomitant obsessive–compulsive disorder and Tourette's syndrome. Archives of General Psychiatry, 51, 73–4.

Kurlan, R. et al. (1990). Neurosurgical treatment of severe obsessive compulsive disorder associated with Tourette's syndrome. Movement Disorders, 5, 152–5.

Robertson, M., et al. (1990). The treatment of Gilles de la Tourette syndrome by limbic leucotomy. Journal of Neurology, Neurosurgery and Psychiatry, 53, 691–4.

Rauch, S.L. et al. (1995). Neurosurgical treatment of Tourette's syndrome: a critical review. Comprehensive Psychiatry, 36 (2), 141–56.

Assessment of Tourette syndrome

Chappell, P.B. et al. (1994). Videotape tic counts in the assessment of Tourette's syndrome: stability, reliability and validity. Journal of the American Academy of Child and Adolescent Psychiatry, 33, 386–93.

Goetz, C.G. et al. (1987) A rating scale for Gilles de La Tourette's syndrome: description, reliability and validity data. Neurology, 37, 1542–4.

Harcherik, D.F. et al. (1984). A new instrument for clinical studies of Tourette syndrome: A preliminary report. Journal of the American Academy of Child Psychiatry, 23, 153–60.

Leckman, J.F., Riddle, M.A., and Hardin, M.T. (1989). The Yale Global Tic Severity Scale: initial testing of a clinician-rated scale of tic severity. Journal of the American Academy of Child and Adolescent Psychiatry, 28, 566–73.

Robertson, M.M. and Eapen, V. (1996). The national hospital interview schedule for the assessment of Gilles de la Tourette syndrome. *International Journal of Methods in Psychiatric Research*, **6**, 203–26.

Shapiro, A.K. and Shapiro, E. (1984). Controlled study of pirotide vs Placebo in Tourette's syndrome. *Journal of the American Academy of Child Psychiatry*, **23**, 161–73 (*Shapiro Tourette Syndrome Severity Scale*)

Walkup, J.T. *et al.* (1992). The validity of instruments measuring tic severity in Tourette's syndrome. *Journal of the American Academy of Child and Adolescent Psychiatry* **31**, 472–7 (*The Hopkins Motor and Vocal Tic Scale*).

General reviews

Hyde, T.M. and Weinberger, D.R. (1995). Tourette's syndrome. a model neuropsychiatric disorder [clinical conference]. *Journal of the American Medical Association*, **273**, 498–501.

Kurlan, R. (1989). Tourette's syndrome: current concepts. *Neurology*, **39**, 1625–30.

Leckman, J.F., Peterson, B.S., and Anderson, G.M. (1997). Pathogenesis of Tourette's syndrome. *Journal of Child Psychology and Psychiatry*, **38**, 119–42.

Robertson, M.M. (1989). The Gilles de la Tourette syndrome: The current status. *British Journal of Psychiatry*, **154**, 147–69.

Robertson, M.M. (1991). Obsessional disorder and the Gilles de la Tourette sydnrome. *Current Opinion in Paedatrics*, 615–23.

Robertson, M.M. (1992). Self-injurious behavior and Tourette syndrome. *In*: T.N. Chase, A.J. Friedhoff, and D.J. Cohen (eds), *Tourette syndrome: genetics, neurobiology and treatment, advances in neurology*, Vol 58, pp.105–14. Raven Press, New York.

Robertson, M.M. (1994). Annotation: Gilles de la Tourette syndrome—an update. *Journal of Child Psychology and Psychiatry*, **35**, 597–611.

Robertson, M.M. (1996). D2 be or not to be? *Nature Medicine*, **2**, 1076–7.

Robertson, M.M. and Boardman, J. (1996). Tourette's syndrome in the year 2000. *Australian and New Zealand Journal of Psychiatry*, **30**, 749–59.

Shapiro, A.K. and Shapiro, E.S. (1982). Tourette syndrome; history and present status. *In*: A.J. Friedhoff, and T.N. Chase (eds): *The Gilles de la Tourette syndrome*, Advances in Neurology, Vol 35, pp 17–23. Raven Press, New York.

Books

Bruun, R.D. and Bruun, B. (1994). A *mind of its own. Tourette's syndrome: a story and a guide.* Oxford University Press, New York.

Chase, T.N., Friedhoff, A.J., and Cohen, D.J. (eds) (1992). Tourette syndrome: genetics, neurobiology, and treatment. *Advances in Neurology,* **58**, Raven Press, New York

Cohen, D.J., Bruun, R.D., and Leckman, J.F. (eds) (1988). *Tourette's syndrome & tic disorders.* John Wiley and Sons, New York.

Comings, D.E. (1990). *Tourette syndrome and human behavior.* Hope Press, Duarte, California.

Kurlan, R. (ed.) (1993). *Handbook of Tourette's syndrome and related tic and behavioral disorders.* Marcel Dekker, New York.

Robertson, M.M. and Eapen, V. (eds) (1995). *Movement and allied disorders in childhood.* John Wiley and Sons, Chichester.

Sacks, O. (1986). *The man who mistook his wife for a hat.* Picador, London.

Sacks, O. (1995). *An anthropologist on Mars.* Vintage Books (Random House Inc), New York.

Shapiro, A.K. *et al.* (1978). *Gilles de la Tourette syndrome.* Raven Press, New York.

Shapiro, A.K. *et al.* (1988). *Gilles de la Tourette syndrome* (2nd edition) Raven Press, New York.

Tourette syndrome around the World

Abuzzahab, F.E. and Anderson, F.G. (1973). Gilles de la Tourette syndrome; International Registry, *Minnesota Medicine*, **56**, 492–6.

Attah Johnson, F.Y. (1996). Gilles de la Tourette syndrome in Papua New Guinea. *Papua New Guinea Medical Journal*, **38** (4) 55–60.

Bai, C.H. and Han-Quin, L.F. (1983). Tourette syndrome: report of 19 cases. *Chinese Medical Journal*, **96**, 45–8.

Berthier, M.L., Bayes, A., and Tolosa, E.S. (1993). Magnetic resonance imaging in patients with concurrent Tourette's disorder and Asperger's syndrome. *Journal of the American Academy of Child and Adolescent Psychiatry*, **32**, 633–9 (Spain).

Cardoso, F., Veado, C.C.M., and de Oliviera, J.T. (1996). A Brazilian cohort of patients with Tourette's syndrome. *Journal of Neurology, Neurosurgery and Psychiatry*, **60**, 209–12.

Chee, K-Y., and Sachdev, P. (1994). The clinical features of Tourette's disorder: an Australian study using a structured interview schedule. *Australian and New Zealand Journal of Psychiatry*, **28**, 313–18.

Cheng, Y. and Jiang, D.H. (1990). Therapeutic effect of inosine in Tourette syndrome and its possible mechanism of action. *Chung Hua Shen Ching Ching Shen Ko Tsa Chih*, **23**, 90–3; 126–27 (China).

Damjanovic, A., Kostic, V.S., and Sternic, N. (1992). Gilles de la Tourette syndrome. *Srp Arth Celok Lek,*. **120,** 197–202. (Serbo-Croatia)

Eapen, V. and Robertson, M.M. (1992). Gilles de la Tourette syndrome—a case report from Guyana in South America. *Behavioural Neurology* **5**, 39–41.

Eapen, V. and Srinath, S. (1992) Gilles de la Tourette syndrome in India. *Psychological Reports*, **70**, 1–2.

Eapen, V. and Robertson, M.M. (1995). Gilles de la Tourette syndrome in Malta—psychopathology in a multiply affected pedigree. *The Arab Journal of Psychiatry*, **6**, 113–18.

El-Assra, A. (1987). A case of Gilles de la Tourette's syndrome in Saudi Arabia. *British Journal of Psychiatry*, **151**, 397–8.

Ellison, R.M. (1964). Gilles de la Tourette's syndrome. *Medical Journal of Australia*, **1**, 153–5.

Fontanari, J.L. and Vaitses, V.D.C. (1896). Sindrome de Gilles de la Tourette e multiplos tiques-estudo clinico de 15 casos e revisao da literatura. *Neurobiologica*, (Recife) **49**, 109–28.

Fulton, W.A., Shady, G.A., and Champion, L.M. (1988). An evaluation of Tourette syndrome and medication use in Canada. *Neurosciences and Biobehavioural Reviews*, **12** (3–4), 251–4.

Gericke, G.S. *et al.* (1995) Increased chromosomal breakage in Tourette syndrome predicts the possibility of variable multiple gene involvement in spectrum phenotypes: preliminary findings and hypothesis. *American Journal of Medical Genetics,*, **60** (5), 444–7 (South Africa).

Golfeto, J.H., Loureiro, S.R., and Ribeiro, M.V. (1988). O sindrome de Gilles de la Tourette: estudo de um caso (Gilles de la Tourette syndrome: a case report), *Neurobiologica,,* **51**, 189–202 (Brazil).

Groot, M.H. de, Bardwell, B. (1970). A case of Gilles de la Tourette's syndrome occurring in New Zealand. *Australia and New Zealand Journal of Psychiatry*, **4**, 155–8.

Hundervadt, L. (1986). Kronisk multiple tics og Gilles de la Tourettes syndrome. *Tidsskr Nor Laegeforen,,* **106**, 207–10 (Norway).

Hussain, M. (1992). Gilles de la Tourette's syndrome. *Journal of the Pakistan Medical Association*, **42** 910, 248–9.

Kano, Y. *et al.* (1988). Tourette's disorder coupled with infantile autism: a prospective study of two boys. *Japanese Journal of Psychiatry and Neurology*, **42** (1), 49–57 (Japan).

Lechin, F. *et al.* (1982). On the use of clonidine and thioproperazine in a woman with Gilles de la Tourette disease. *Biological Psychiatry,,* **17**, 103–8 (Venezuela).

Lees, A.J. *et al.* (1984). A clinical study of the Gilles de la Tourette syndrome in the United Kingdom. *Journal of Neurology, Neurosurgery, and Psychiatry*, **47**, 1–8.

Lieh Mak, F. *et al.* (1982). Tourette syndrome in the Chinese: a follow-up of 15 cases. *In*: A.J. Friedhoff, and T.N. Chase, (eds), *Gilles de la Tourette syndrome*, 281–4. Raven Press, New York.

Lieh Mak, F., Luk, S.L., and Leung, L. (1979). Gilles de la Tourette's syndrome: report of five cases in the Chinese. *British Journal of Psychiatry*, **134**, 630–4.

Micheli, F., Gatto, M., and Gershanik, O. (1995). Gilles de la Tourette syndrome: clinical features of 75 cases from Argentina. *Behavioural Neurology*, **8**, 75–80.

Min, S.K. and Lee, H. (1986). A clinical study of Gilles de la Tourette's syndrome in Korea. *British Journal of Psychiatry*, **149**, 644–7.

Nishida, H., Shinbo, Y., and Motomura, H. (1994). A study of pathogenesis and symptoms of Tourette's syndrome—mainly on the importance of 'startle reflex' through Latah reaction. *Seishin Shinkeigaku Zasshi*, **96**, (1) 26–47 (Japan).

Nomoto, F. and Machiyama, Y. (1990). An epidemiological study of tics. *Japanese Journal of Psychiatry and Neurology*, **44**, 649–55.

Nomura, Y. and Segawa, M. (1982). Tourette syndrome in Oriental children: clinical and pathophysiological considerations. *In*: A.J.

Friedhoff and T.N. Chase (eds) *Gilles de la Tourette syndrome*, Advances in Neurology, Vol 35, pp.277–80. Raven Press, New York (Japan).

Nomura, Y., Kita, M., Segawa, M. (1992). Social adaptation of Tourette syndrome families in Japan. *In*: T.N. Chase, A.J. Friedhoff, and D.J. Cohen (eds): *Tourette syndrome: genetics, neurobiology and treatment, advances in neurology*, Vol 58, pp.323–32. Raven Press, New York.

Perera, H.V. (1975). Two cases of Gilles de la Tourette's syndrome treated with haloperidol. *British Journal of Psychiatry*, **127**, 324–6. (Sri Lanka)

Prabhakan, N. (1970). A case of Gilles de la Tourette's syndrome with some observations on aetiology and treatment. *British Journal of Psychiatry*, **116**, 539–41 (India).

Prata, G. and Masson, O. (1985). Short term therapy of a child with Gilles de la Tourette's syndrome. *Journal of Family Therapy*, **7**, 315–32.

Rabey, J.M. *et al.* (1993). Decreased dopamine uptake into platelet storage granules in Gilles de la Tourette syndrome. *Biological Psychiatry*, **38**, 112–15 (Israel).

Regeur, L. (1992). Clinical evaluation and pharmacological treatment of Gilles de la Tourette's syndrome and other hyperkinesias. *Acta Neurologica Scandinavica*, Suppl, **137**, 48–50 (Denmark).

Robertson, M.M. and Trimble, M.R. (1991). Gilles de la Tourette syndrome in the Middle East: report of a cohort and a multiply affected large pedigree. *British Journal of Psychiatry*, **158**, 416–19.

Robertson, M.M. *et al.* (1994). Tourette's syndrome in New Zealand. A postal survey. *British Journal of Psychiatry*, **164**, 263–6.

Sandor, P. *et al.* (1990). Tourette syndrome: a follow-up study. *Journal of Clinical Psychopharmacology*, **10**, 197–9 (Canada).

Shenken, L. (1980). A case of the Gilles de la Tourette syndrome. *New Zealand Medical Journal*, **668**, 234–5 (New Zealand).

Silvestri, R. *et al.* (1994). Serotoninergic agents in the treatment of Gilles de la Tourette's syndrome. *Acta Neurologica Napoli*, **16** (1–2), 58–63. (Italy)

Smirnov, A. (1990). Clinical variability of the Gilles de la Tourette syndrome: the heterogeneity of the classical syndrome. *Zh Nevropatol Psikhiatr Im S S Korsakova*, **90**, 61–6 (Russia).

Temlett, J.A. *et al.* (1995). Misdiagnosis of Gilles de la Tourette syndrome (letter). *South African Medical Journal*, **85** (3), 187–88 (South Africa).

Teoh, J.I. (1974). Gilles de la Tourette's syndrome: a study of the treatment of six cases by mass negative practice and with haloperidol. *Singapore Medical Journal*, **15** (2) 139–46.

Van Woerkom, T.C., Roos, R.A., and van Dijk, J.G. (1994). Altered attentional processing of background stimuli in Gilles de la Tourette syndrome: a study in auditory event-related potentials evoked in an oddball paradigm. *Acta Neurologica Scandinavica*, **90** (2), 116–23 (Netherlands).

Wong, C.K. and Lau, J.T.F. (1993). Psychiatric morbidity in a Chinese primary school in Hong Kong. *Australian and New Zealand Journal of Psychiatry*, **27**, 666–72.

Yordanova, J., Dumais-Huber, C., and Rothenberger, A. (1996). Coexistence of tics and hyperactivity in children: no additive effect at the psychophysiological level. *International Journal of Psychophysiology*, **21**, 121–33 (Germany).

Zelnik, N. (1992). Early developmental aspects of Tourette syndrome. *Harefuah*, **122**(5), 301–04. (Israel)

Zhisheng, L. Z *et al.* (1996). A neuropsychological analysis and its relations with plasma prolactin level in children with Tourette's syndrome. *Chinese Journal of Pediatrics*, **34** (2), 84–7.

Appendix 3
List of Tourette Syndrome Associations and international contacts*

Argentina
Oscar Gershanik M.D.
Fundacion Thomson
La Rioja 951
Capital Federal
Buenos Aires, Argentina

Lic. Luisa Osdoba
Donato Alvarez 205
Cap. Fed (1406) 2°C
Buenos Aires, Argentina

Frederico Micheli M.D.
Universidad de Buenos Aires
Facultad de Medicina
Dept Neurologia
Hospital de Clinicas
Jose de San Martin
Cordoba 2361
Buenos Aires
Tel + 54-1-811-3076

Australia
Tourette Syndrome Association
Of Victoria Inc.
34 Jackson Street
Toorak 3142, Victoria, Australia
Tel. + 03-9828-7218
Fax: + 03-9826-9054

Tourette Syndrome Association
of Australia
PO Box 1173
Maroubra, NSW 2035, Australia
Tel/Fax: + 02-9311-2745

Western Australian Tourette
Syndrome Organisation, Inc.
Paul M. Smith, President
Neurological Lotteries House
320 Rokeby Road
Subaco W.A. 6008 Australia
Tel. + 61-893-883-486
Fax: + 61-893-821-149

Austria
Maria Stamenkovic M.D.
Schindler Shird M.D.
Department of General
Psychiatry
Vienna University Hospital of
Psychiatry
Wahringergurtel 18–20
A-1090 Vienna, Austria
Tel. + 43-140-400-3526
Fax: + 43-140-400-3560

Belgium
Gilles de la Tourette
Vera Casier Cassimon, Pres.
(Flemish)
Vlaamse Vereniging Gilles de la
Tourette
v.z.w. - J. Nauwelaertstraat, 7
2210 Wijnegen, Belgium
Tel. + 32-3-354-3669
Fax: + 32-3-353-6791

Patricia Seminerio (French)
17 Avenue Bel Horizon
1301 Bierges/Wavre, Belgium
Tel/Fax: + 32-10-41-7052

* Compiled September 1997

Brazil
Euripedes C. Miguel M.D., Ph.D.
PROTOC do IPQ-HCFMUSP
Rua Ovidio Pires de Campos,
s/n°-s.4021
05403-010 Sao Paulo, SP, Brazil
Tel/Fax: + 5-11-853-3531

Christina de Luca/Maura de
Carvallo
R Bras Cardoso 201
Sao Paulo – Brazil
Cep. 04510-030
Fax: 5511-822-0023

Bulgaria
Dr Dimiter Terziev
Child Psychiatric Clinic
33, Prohlada Street
16169 – Sofia, Bulgaria

Canada
Ts Foundation of Canada
Rosie Wartecker, Executive
Director
194 Jarvis St, Suite 206
Toronto, Ontario M5B 2B7
Tel. + 416-861-8398
Fax: + 416-861-2472
Toll Free No: 1-800-361-3120

Vancouver Island Tourette
Syndrome Chapter
Judy Rogers
c/o 805–510 Marsett Place
Victoria, BC V82-7J1
Tel. 604/658-0506

Chile
Carla Hendee
Casilla 342
Maipu, Chile, S.A.

China
Dr Liu Zhisheng
Department of Neurology
Guangzhou Children's Hospital

No. 318 Renmin Zhong Road
Guangzhou 510120, China
Tel. + (86-20) 8188-6332
ext. 5702
Fax: + (86-10) 8186-1650

Zhang Shi Ji, M.D.
Beijing Child and Adolescent
Mental Health Center
5, Ankang Avenue, De Sheng
Men Wai
Beijing, China 100088
Tel. + (86-10) 6425-5034

Colombia
Maria Alicia Irequi
Apartado Ae'reo 250914
Bogota, Colombia, S.A.
Tel. + 57-1-310-6616

Croatia
Dubravka Kocijan
Clinic Hospital Dubrava
Aleja Izvidsca 6
1000 Zagreb, Croatia

Cyprus
Angela Charalambous
Adrocleous 15
Flat 102
Nicosia, Cyprus
Tel. + 003572-466750
Fax: + 003572-362488

Denmark
Dansk Tourette Forening
Kjeld Christensen, President
Prestehusene 31
DK 2820 Denmark
Tel. + 45-43-96-57-09

Kirsten Kristensen
Sollerodvej 7B
DK 2840 Holte
Denmark
Tel. + 45-45-80-07-53

Ecuador
Vicente Maldonado
Lizardo Garcia
328 y 6 du Diciembre
Quito, Eduador

Finland
Ella Niemi
Project Secretary
The Finnish MS-Society
Seppalantie 90, Masku
PO Box 15, SF-21251 Masku,
Finland
Tel. + 358-21-439-2111
Fax: + 358-21-439-2112

Kenneth Carlberg
Manager, Kurscentret Hogsand
FS 10 820 Hogsand, Finland
Tel. + 358-19-244-3800
Fax: + 358-19-244-3740

France
Aftoc-Tourette
Bridget Haardt
17, rue Paule Borghese
F 92200 Neuilly Sur Seine
France
Tel. + 33-1-47-38-29-08
Fax: + 33-1-47-38-18-10

Germany
Tourette Gesellschaft
Deutschland
Prof. Dr. A. Rothenberger, Vice
President
Universitat Gottingen
Abteilung fur Kinder-und
Jugendypsychiatrie
von-Siebold-Str. 5
D 37075 Gottingen, Germany

Karl Joseph
Stolting Hof 1
D 30 455 Hannover
Germany
Tel. + 49-511-486-262

Johannes Hebebrand, M.D.
Dept. Of Child & Adolescent
Psychiatry
Philipps University of Marburg
Hans-Sachs-Str. 6
D-35033, Marburg, Germany
Tel. + 49-6421-286-466
Fax: + 49-6421-283-056
E-mail:
jonas@mvkjp2.kjp.uni.marburg.de

Great Britain
Tourette Syndrome (UK)
Association
Paul Smith, National
Coordinator
Iain Steedman, General Secretary
1st Floor Offices, Old Bank
Chambers
London Road, Crowborough
East Sussex, TN6 2TT, UK
Tel. + 44-1892-669-151
Fax: + 44-1892-663-649
E-mail: 101667.3131
@compuserve.com

Chris Mansley
Watling Street, Fulwood
Preston, Lancs, U.K.

Greece
Dr Anastasia Koumoula
Child Psychiatric Hospital
Garefi 4
N Psychiko
Greece
Tel. + 301-6773442
Fax: + 301-6773445

Hong Kong
Michael and Hava Udalevich
Baguio Villa BLK 46 (19FL)
550 Victoria Road
Pok Fulam
Hong Kong

Tel. + 852-2550-2594
Fax: + 852-2875-3416
E-mail:
MRYU@NETVIGATOR.COM

Professor Felice Lieh Mak
Department of Psychiatry
University of Hong Kong
Hong Kong
China
Fax: 00852 2855 1345

Hungary
Dr Attila Nemeth MD. PhD,
President of Hungarian
Obsessive-Compulsive
Association, Ilaynal Imre
University of Health Services
Department of Psychiatry
POB1,
Budapest
Hungary 1281
Tel: + 361-176-0922
Fax: + 361-393-0281

Iceland
Tourette Samtokin a Islandi
Elisabeth K. Magnusdottir,
President
Postholf 3128
IS 123 Reykjavik, Iceland
Tel. + 354-588-8581
Fax: + 354-551-4580

India
Mrs Jaishri Iyer
No. 154, S.F.S. (208), G.K.V.K.
Post
Yelahanka, Bangalore-560065,
India
Tel. + 91-80-846-2392

Dr Shoba Srinath
National Institute of Mental
Health and Neurosciences
Deemed University

Department of Psychiatry
P.O. Box No 2900
Bangalore 560 029
India
Tel. + 91-80-664-2121
Fax: + 91-80-663-1830

Iraq
Ali Maziad Abd. Al. Azeez
P.O.Box 46114
Postal Code 12506
Al-Mustansiriya University
Baghdad, Iraq
Tel. (H) + 964-425-7119
(W) + 964-1-541-5591

Ireland
Tourette Syndrome Association
of Ireland
39, Elderwood Road
Palmerstown, Dublin 20

Mrs Una Finucane
29 Granville Road
Dun Laoghaire
Co Dublin, Eire
Tel. + 353-1-285-2193
Fax: + 353-1-808-2578 (c/o
Brendan)

Israel
TSA of Israel
P.O. Box 7018
Ramat Gan, Israel 52170
Tel. + 972-9-740-8478

Nahum Muskat
Fax: + 00972-6-341466

Italy
Prof. Michele Zappella
Department of Child
Neuropsychiatry
Via Mattioli 10
53100 Siena, Italy

Japan
Masako Kaji
Dystonia Support Group of Japan
2-1917 Sencho
OHTSU-City Shiga 520, Japan
Tel. + 81-775-33-0297
Fax: + 81-775-33-0297

Dr Masaya Segawa/Dr Yoshiko
Nomura
Segawa Neurological Clinic for
Children
2–8 Surugadai, Kanda
Chiyoda-Ku, Tokyo 101, Japan
Tel. + 81-3-294-0371
Fax: + 81-3-294-0290

Mr and Mrs J. Dando
Yagoto Shataku East A401
4–17 Yamate Dori, Showa Ku
Nagoya Shi, Aichi 466, Japan
Tel. + 052-834-4670

Korea (South)
Professor Michael Hong
Seoul National Univ. Children's
Hospital
Div. of Child & Adolescent
Psychiatry
28 Yongon-Dong, Chongno-gu
Seoul 110-744, Korea
Tel. + 82-2-760-3647
Fax: + 82-2-747-5774

Soo Churl Cho, M.D.
Dept. of Neuropsychiatry
College of Medicine
Souel National University
#28 Yeongun-Dong, Chongro
Seoul 110-744, Korea

Young-Suk Paik, M.D.
Wonkwang Univ.
Neuropsychiatric Hospital
144–23 Dongsan-dong, Iksan

Chonpuk 570-060, South Korea
Tel. + (653) 840-6005
Fax: + (653) 840-6069

Libya
Dr A. Alsanossi
P.O. Box 20240, Sebha, Libya

Lithuania
Valmantas Budrys, MD, Ph.D.
Vilnius University Hospital
Santariskiu Klinikos
Santariskiu gatve 2
LT 2600 Vilnius, Lithuania

Netherlands
Stichting Gilles de la Tourette
Hans Eijsacher, President
de Schans 20
3144 ET Maassleus
The Netherlands
Tel. + 31-10-591-5278

Ben B.J.M. van de Wetering,
MD, Ph.D.
Dept. of Psychiatry – Outpatient
Service
Univ. Hospital Rotterdam-
Dijkzigt
Dr Molewaterplein 40
3015 GD Rotterdam, The
Netherlands
Tel. + 31-10-463-5871
Fax: + 31-10-463-5867

New Zealand
David and Caroline Ashby
258 Kennedy Road
Napier
New Zealand

Norway
H.C.A. Melbye, International
Contact
Munkerudasen 33

N 1165 Oslo, Norway
Tel. & Fax: + 47-22-285-043

Norsk Tourette Forening
Tom A. Wulff, President
Brolandsveien 19B
N-0980 Oslo, Norway
Tel. + 47-22-216-506
Fax: + 47-22-109-921
E-Mail: tomwulff@online.no

Pakistan
Professor Musarrat Hussain
Department of Psychiatry
Jinnah Postgraduate Medical
Centre (JPMC)
Karachi, 75510
Pakistan
Tel. + 92-21-52003346
Fax: + 92-21-5676023

Papua New Guinea
Dr Felix Attah Johnson
Associate Professor of Psychiatry
University of Papua New Guinea
PO Box 5623
Boroko, NCD
Papua New Guinea
Tel: 00-1-675-324-8451
Fax: 00-1-675-325-4935

Paraguay
Jose Raul Torres Kirmser
Avenida General Santos u-330
Asuncion, Paraguay

Peru
Norka Lopez
La Chalana 225
La Molina
Lima 12, Peru
Fax: + 51-1-479-0430

Association Sindrome de
Tourette del Peru

Luisa Fernanda L. de Romana,
Gen. Sec.
Las Golondrinas #390, DPTO
'A' 2-00
Lima 27, Peru
Fax: + 51-1-224-7567

Poland
Kalina Michalkiewicz
ul. Plocka 12 m 51
01-231 Warszawa, Poland

Puerto Rico
Flora Santiago
Esmeralda #52, Villa Blanca
Caguas, P.R. 00725

Russia
Janna Baranovskaja
Tel. + 7-095-267-7083 (office)
+ 7-095-218-6566 (home)
Fax: + 7-501-940-2310

South Africa
Southern Africa Tourette
Syndrome Institute (SATSI)
Johan van der Westhuizen,
President
228 Oak Avenue
Ferndale, 2194
South Africa
Tel. + 27-11-886-6353

Izelda Pelser
Neurogenetic Clinic
Institute for Pathology Building
P.O. Box 2034
Pretoria 0001, South Africa
Tel. + 27-12-324-5060
Fax: + 27-12-323-2788

George S. Gericke, MBChB,
MMed.
Prof. and Head, Dept. of Human
Genetics and Developmental
Biology

University of Pretoria
P.O. Box 2034, Pretoria 0001
Republic of South Africa
Tel. + 012-329-1111
Fax: + 012-329-1343

Ellen Nortje
P.O. Box 26529
Hout Bay 7872
Cape Province, South Africa
Tel. + 27-21-790-2502

Professor James Temlett
University of Witwatersrand
Department of Neurology
7 York Road
Parktown
Johannesburg 2193
Republic of South Africa
Tel: 00-27-11-488-4433
Fax: 00-27-11-488-4454

Spain
Eduardo Tolosa, M.D.
Neurology Service, Hospital
Clinico
1 Provincial de Barcelona
Villaroel, 170-08036 Barcelona
Spain
Tel. + 34-3-227-5400
Fax: + 34-3-227-5454

Jaime Diaz Guzman, M.D.
Servicio de Neurologia
Hospital Universitario Doce de
Octubre
Carretera de Andalucia Km
5,400
28041 Madrid, Spain

Sweden
The Swedish Tourette
Association
c/o Ulf Christansson
Soerkroken 2, S-440 74

Hjaelteby
Sweden
Tel. + 46-304-678-130
Fax: + 46-304-678-130
Email: ulf.c@kpab.se

Svensk Tourette Forening
Eva Helberg, President
Vindheimsgatan 12
S 752 24 Uppsala, Sweden
Tel. + 46-18-552-544

Switzerland
Tourette Gesellschaft Schweiz
Guido Hilfiker, President
Dorfstrasse 64
CH 8912 Obfelden, Switzerland
Tel. + 41-1-760-0265

Jurg Timm
Tel. + 41-71-722-2506

Gigi Kundert
Tel. + 41-52-376-1077

Taiwan
Shu-Yin Chen
No. 7–1, Lane 49, Ming Chung
Street
Hsin Chung City, Taipei Hsien
Taiwan, R.O.C.
Fax: + 886-2-993-4984

Thailand
Dr Niphon Poungvarin
Professor of Neurology
Department of Medicine
Faculty of Medicine Siriraj
Mahidol University
Prannock Road
Bangkok 10700
Thailand
Tel: 00-2-411-1103
Fax: 00-662-412-5994

Dr Spain Une Anong
Department of Psychaitry
Ramathibodi Hospital
Mahidol University
Rama VI Road
Bangkok 10400
Thailand
Tel: 00-662-245-5704
Fax: 00-662-246-2123

Turkey
M. Yanki Yazgan M.D.
Marmara University
Faculty of Psychiatry
Altunizade, Istanbul
Turkey 81190
Tel. + 90-216-332-2553

United Arab Emirates
Dr Valsamma Eapen
Assistant Professor in Child
Psychiatry
UAE University
Faculty of Medicine and Health
Sciences

PO Box 17666
Al Ain
United Arab Emirates
Tel: 00-971-3-669584
Fax: 00-971-3-657649

United States of America
Tourette Syndrome Association
42-40 Bell Boulevard
Bayside
NY 11631-2820
USA
Tel: 00-1-718-224-2999
Fax: 00-1-718-279-9596
E-mail:
Tourette@!X.Netcom.com

Zimbabwe
Peter Perry
P.O. Box M187
Mabelreign, Harare
Zimbabwe
Tel. and Fax; + 263-4-741-884

Index